Bebiana Calisto Bernardo

Risk Factors for Sexual Transmission of HIV in Angolan Pregnant Women

Bebiana Calisto Bernardo

Risk Factors for Sexual Transmission of HIV in Angolan Pregnant Women

Female Sexuality and HIV

Imprint
Any brand names and product names mentioned in this book are subject to trademark, brand or patent protection and are trademarks or registered trademarks of their respective holders. The use of brand names, product names, common names, trade names, product descriptions etc. even without a particular marking in this work is in no way to be construed to mean that such names may be regarded as unrestricted in respect of trademark and brand protection legislation and could thus be used by anyone.

Cover image: www.ingimage.com

This book is a translation from the original published under ISBN 978-613-9-61457-8.

Publisher:
Sciencia Scripts
is a trademark of
Dodo Books Indian Ocean Ltd. and OmniScriptum S.R.L publishing group

120 High Road, East Finchley, London, N2 9ED, United Kingdom
Str. Armeneasca 28/1, office 1, Chisinau MD-2012, Republic of Moldova, Europe
Printed at: see last page
ISBN: 978-620-7-68388-8

Table of contents:

Chapter 1	7
Chapter 2	16
Chapter 3	17
Chapter 4	24
Chapter 5	35

RISK FACTORS FOR SEXUAL TRANSMISSION OF HIV IN ANGOLAN PREGNANT WOMEN

BEBIANA CALISTO BERNARDO

RECIFE - PE

2011

I dedicate it to my children:
Cintia, Arieh and Noemia who have been with me
on this difficult road.

ACKNOWLEDGMENTS

To Professors Ricardo Ximenes and Heloisa Ramos Lacerda for the opportunity, support and teachings,

I would like to thank Professor Vera Magalhaes, representing all the professors of the Postgraduate Program in Tropical Medicine.

Thanks to Valter Leite and Alice for their invaluable support and dedication.

To all my doctoral colleagues.

To my dear friends Claudia Zírpolli, Valeria de Albuquerque, Joao José do Amaral (Duda) and Luiza Menezes, who closely participated in my days of success and sadness.

SUMMARY

In order to estimate the frequency of risk factors for sexual transmission of HIV in pregnant women in the public health network in Luanda, and to verify their association with HIV/AIDS, a case-control study was carried out involving 1092 women (273 cases and 819 controls) from August 2007 to December 2009. This study comprises three articles:

1. Association between demographic, socioeconomic and political factors and the sexual transmission of HIV in pregnant women. Demographic factors: age, place of residence and ethnicity; Socioeconomic factors: occupation, income, type of housing, water and energy supply and ownership of household goods; Political factors: having experienced war showed a statistically significant association with HIV.

2. Association between cultural factors and the sexual transmission of HIV in pregnant women - Having two or more previous marital relationships, being a victim of psychological violence, living in a polygamous union and taking the initiative for an affective relationship had a higher chance of HIV infection.

3. Association between behavioral factors and the sexual transmission of HIV in pregnant women - The serology of the partner, high number of partners, lack of condom use and sexual relations under the influence of alcohol characterized the women while for the partners, age, schooling, frequenting the barbershop, alcohol use and length of relationship were the behavioral aspects associated with HIV.

The association between HIV and age suggests an increased prevalence of infection from the age of 30 onwards and consequently under-reporting in younger women, implying that women's health policies should target this group and encourage voluntary HIV testing before pregnancy. Socio-economic status showed no clear association with HIV infection, suggesting a double pattern, thus highlighting the complexity of the network of determinants of infection. Cultural barriers can make it difficult for society to be more open to sexual and reproductive health. Behavioral factors suggest the existence of asymmetrical relationships, lack of adherence to condom use and little space for women to negotiate safe sex.

Key Words: HIV, sexual transmission, pregnant women, risk factors

PRESENTATION

Based on the assumption that the knowledge, values and practices of a population may differ in different regions, because they reflect their culture, tradition and life history, it is accepted that the risk factors for the Acquired Immunodeficiency Virus - HIV present themselves in a peculiar way among individuals in the same society as well as in different regions of the world (COSTA JF., 1998; GONCALVES EH, GUILHEM D. 2003; GUILHEM D. 2005; MAIA, C.; GUILHEM, D. ; FREITAS, D. 2008; STRAZZA ET AL., 2003). Considering this principle, it is believed that the socio-economic, cultural and civil war peculiarities may make Angolan women more vulnerable to HIV/AIDS (DUFFY, 2005; FRASER, 2005; PRATA, B. N; VAHIDNIA, F; MONTEIRO, S 2009; WHO, 1999). Given the scarcity of local studies on women's vulnerability to HIV, this study was proposed with the aim of contributing to the definition of policies that promote knowledge, changes in behavior and attitudes that increase women's risk of becoming infected with HIV. The main objective of this study was to identify the prevalence of risk factors (socio-economic, demographic, political, cultural and behavioral) and to determine their association with the sexual transmission of HIV in Angolan women living in the metropolitan region of Luanda - Republic of Angola. This study includes a brief review of the literature, the methodology used and the presentation of the results in the form of articles distributed as follows:

Article1* - Association between demographic, socio-economic and political factors and the sexual transmission of HIV in pregnant women;

Article2* - Association between cultural factors and the sexual transmission of HIV in pregnant women;

Article3* - Association between characteristics and behavioral factors in pregnant women and their partners and the sexual transmission of HIV.

Chapter 1

1- - LITERATURE REVIEW

1.1 - Epidemiological aspects of hiv/aids

HIV infection represents a serious public health problem and the risk factors for its transmissibility have been the subject of studies around the world.

The HIV/AIDS epidemic is a dynamic phenomenon that progressively involves more segments of the population and the way it occurs in different regions of the world depends on individual and collective human behavior (WOOD, 2002). According to world statistics, at the end of 2008 there were around 33.4 million people infected with HIV/AIDS worldwide, with sub-Saharan Africa being the region most affected, with 67% of the total, followed by Asia, with 14%. In the Americas, the countries most affected by the epidemic are the United States of America (USA) and Brazil. According to these estimates, AIDS was the fourth leading cause of death worldwide (UNAIDS, 2009).

In the West, the group initially most affected was men, gay or bisexual, aged between 20 and 49. However, from the 1990s onwards, there was a significant increase in cases among women, which led to the heterosexualization and feminization of HIV.

In Western Europe, at the end of 2006, 35% of new cases affected women and in Eastern Europe this population group accounted for 41% of cases (EUROHIV, 2006). According to the global statistics presented above, of the 33.4 million people infected with HIV in 2008, 15.7% are women, 60% of whom are African women (UNAIDS and WHO, 2009).

On the African continent, the epidemiological profile of HIV from the outset does not associate AIDS with homosexuals, as has been the case in other regions of the world. Since the initial publications, the female population has led the statistics with higher proportions of infection, thus highlighting the heterosexual route as the main form of spread on this continent. According to a report by the United Nations Joint Program, in 1998 the prevalence of HIV in pregnant women reached 40% (Botswana), while there were 3.9 million deaths and eight million orphans (UNAIDS1998). For every 10 new cases in men, 13 women are infected in the same region (UNAIDS-ODM6, 2010). In this region, women are at greater risk of becoming infected with HIV at a younger age than men aged 15 to 24. The sex ratio in this age group is as high as 13 women to 10 men in sub-Saharan Africa as a whole, specifically 20 women to 10 young men in South Africa and 45 women to 10 men in Kenya and Mali (UNAIDS, 2004). This picture reflects the continuously expanding feminization of the AIDS epidemic in the female population in sub-Saharan Africa (UNAIDS, 2004) since the beginning of the epidemic. By 2007, infection in women in Africa represented 61% of adults living with HIV compared to 43% in the Caribbean, 26% in Eastern Europe and Central Asia, and 29% in Asia in that period (UNAIDS, 2007).

In Angola, according to estimates by the Ministry of Health (INLS, 2006), since the first case was registered in 1985, there has been an increase to 7 (12%) thousand cases in 1999, rising to one million cases in 2003. Although the lack of methodologically well-structured studies with consistent data does not allow us to know the real epidemiological situation of HIV/AIDS in Angola, it is known that the seroprevalence of pregnant women in the areas bordering Angola exceeds the overall infection rates recorded in the country (INLS, 2006).

The prevalence of HIV-infected individuals (aged 15-45) is 5.3% in Angola, compared to 4.9% in the People's Republic of Congo, which, like Angola, has been at war since 1997 (THE UNITED NATIONS DEVELOPMENT PROGRAMME, 2007). Comparisons with other African countries in this population group show different results: 19% in South Africa, 20% in Zimbabwe, 23% in Lesotho and 33% in Swaziland (THE UNITED NATIONS DEVELOPMENT PROGRAMME, 2007). This discrepancy prompts some reflections, despite the still limited understanding of the phenomena underlying the wide variation in the prevalence of HIV infection between cities and regions in sub-Saharan Africa (AUVERT et al., 2001). In Angola, there is no effective border control with neighboring countries such as Zambia and Namibia, where the prevalence is around 17.0% and 19.6% respectively (THE UNITED NATIONS DEVELOPMENT PROGRAMME, 2007). However, the supposed unrestricted circulation did not influence the prevalence of infection in Angola. The prevalence observed in Angola and the Congo is low, especially if we consider that the civil war scenario could be linked to a lack of respect for human rights, including sexual violence, as well as generating conditions of extreme poverty that would make it easier to engage in the sex trade as a way of surviving (AMOWITZ et al., 2002). However, although the war was associated with the forced displacement of the population with the interruption of cohesion and social relations that predisposed to promiscuity, inadequate accommodation, as well as the inclusion of a high prevalence of HIV within another population with a lower prevalence of infection, the current epidemiological situation in Angola suggests that the war has led to isolation and difficult access for the Angolan population and has thus restricted the spread of infection (THE JOINT UNITED NATIONS PROGRAMME ON HIV/AIDS, 2006). In other countries, such as Kigali, Rwanda, the experience of war revealed a higher prevalence of HIV among pregnant women in rural areas than the national average for that country (LEROY, et al., 1995).

Among the different possibilities for HIV transmission, the heterosexual route is the most frequent (GUIMARÃES and CASTILHO, 1993; BRITO et al., 2001; RODRIGUES and CASTILHO, 2004). Although the risk factors for HIV transmission do not have a direct causal relationship, it is assumed that the presence of a risk factor in a given group of individuals represents a greater probability of contracting HIV/AIDS, and that the presence of a protective factor has the opposite meaning. The risk factors for HIV transmission include demographic, socioeconomic, political, cultural, behavioral and biological aspects that form a chain of determinations that will ultimately influence the practice of unprotected sex and consequently the transmission of HIV.

1.2 - Contextualization of potential risk factors in the study population

HIV infection in the female population remains high in the sub-Saharan region of Africa (UNAIDS, 2009) where underdevelopment (UNDP, 2006) and culture (KALIPENI, GHOSH, AWIRE-VALHMU, 2007) are peculiarities that can influence the behavior and global statistics of the epidemic.

The heterosexual and feminine character that the epidemic has taken on since the 1990s

(Castilho and Chequer 1997; Castilho et al. 1999; Brasil/ MS, 2000); Fonseca et al. 2000; Parker, 2000; Szwarcwald, 1994; UNAIDS, 1999) has been accentuated in poorer regions such as those on the African continent (UNAIDS, 2004). Although heterosexualization is a condition closely linked to the spread of HIV in sub-Saharan Africa, socio-economic, demographic, political, cultural and behavioural factors (UNAIDS, 1998; UNAIDS, 2004; UNAIDS, 2007; UNAIDS-ODM6, 2010) may explain the prominence of the feminization of this epidemic (Medina, 2001; WHO, 1999). It is believed that Angola, an equally underdeveloped country, has cultural and political particularities with socio-economic and demographic implications that can modify behaviors that place women in a situation of vulnerability to HIV.

Understanding that the investigation of risk factors that determine female vulnerability to sexual transmission of HIV can contribute to the identification of women at greater risk of sexual transmission, it is considered relevant to study these factors in Angola, both because of the relevance of the place of study and because of the possible contribution to supporting measures to control the epidemic. However, epidemiological studies investigating risk factors for infectious diseases have pointed to the involvement of a considerable number of variables due to their multi-causal nature (Fuchs et al, 1996, Victora et al, 1997). According to these authors, the involvement of this diversity of factors in vulnerability to an infectious event requires the construction of a hierarchical theoretical conceptual model in order to allow adequate adjustment of the risk factors; This model relativizes statistical significance, facilitates the interpretation of results and grasps the different levels of determinism (Béria et al, 1993; Fuchs et al, 1996; Víctora, 1997; Olinto, 1998; Petry et al, 2000; Rego, 2001; Carret et al, 2004; Nascimento et al, 2004; Macedo et al, 2007).

According to Víctora (1997), in the construction of this type of model, at the upper levels are the determinants with distal participation which, in the case of the sexual transmission of HIV, are the socio-economic, demographic and political factors; at lower levels are the intermediate variables and, finally, the proximal variables, i.e. those which act more directly on the event. The interrelationships between the levels of determination are called mechanisms or causal chains, which can lead to the development of the event. Each of these chains can be a sufficient cause for the outcome to occur. In this study, the theoretical model of hierarchization includes five levels, as shown schematically in the figure below. However, the most distal level, represented by general socioeconomic and demographic aspects, and the most proximal, consisting of biological characteristics, are not the subject of this study. We chose to focus on the levels where there is the greatest possibility of intervention through public policies. The definition of the different levels and the selection of the variables that make up each of them was based on a broad review of the literature and the model was adapted to the specific reality of Angola. The following are some of the topics that allow the model to be contextualized and better understood in the reality of that country.

Conceptual model for sexual transmission of HIV in women

Figure 1 - Conceptual model for sexual transmission of HIV in women

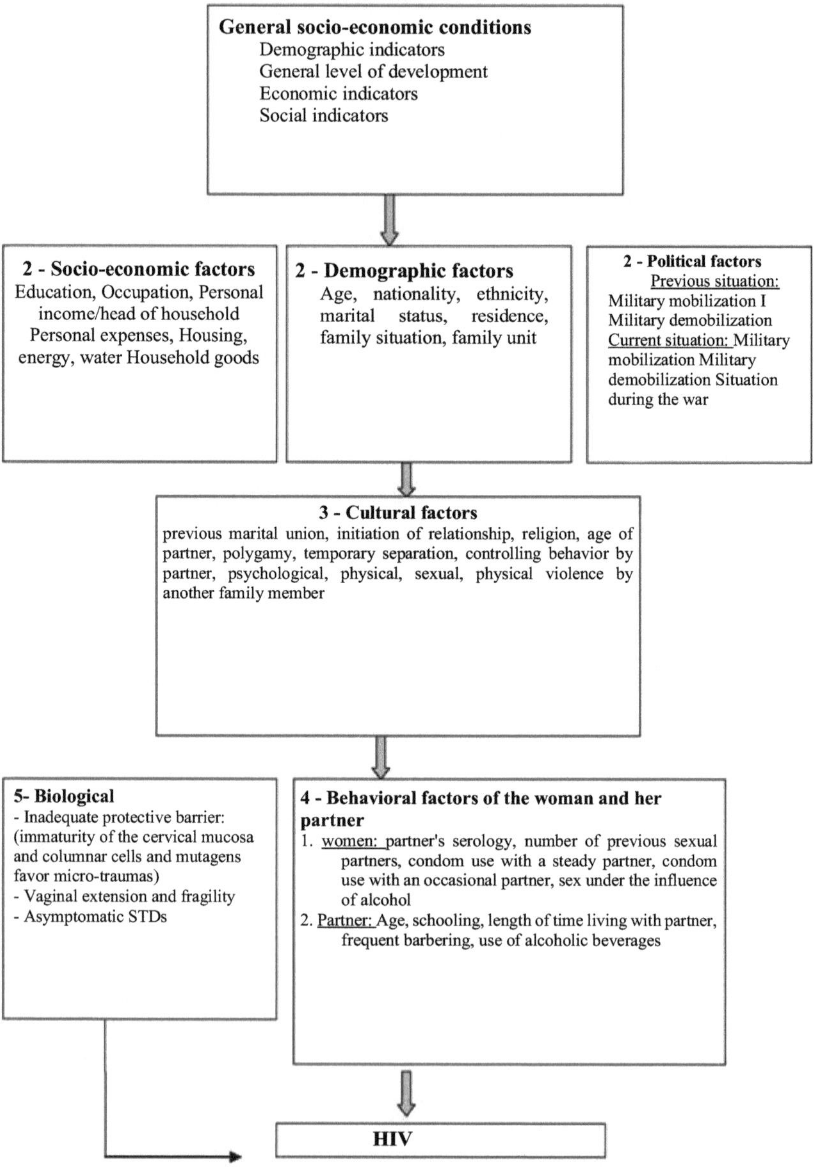

General socio-economic conditions
Demographic indicators
General level of development
Economic indicators
Social indicators

2 - Socio-economic factors
Education, Occupation, Personal income/head of household
Personal expenses, Housing, energy, water Household goods

2 - Demographic factors
Age, nationality, ethnicity, marital status, residence, family situation, family unit

2 - Political factors
Previous situation: Military mobilization I Military demobilization
Current situation: Military mobilization Military demobilization Situation during the war

3 - Cultural factors
previous marital union, initiation of relationship, religion, age of partner, polygamy, temporary separation, controlling behavior by partner, psychological, physical, sexual, physical violence by another family member

5- Biological
- Inadequate protective barrier: (immaturity of the cervical mucosa and columnar cells and mutagens favor micro-traumas)
- Vaginal extension and fragility
- Asymptomatic STDs

4 - Behavioral factors of the woman and her partner
1. women: partner's serology, number of previous sexual partners, condom use with a steady partner, condom use with an occasional partner, sex under the influence of alcohol
2. Partner: Age, schooling, length of time living with partner, frequent barbering, use of alcoholic beverages

HIV

1.2.1 - **Angola's socio-economic situation**

Angola's economic situation has been characterized by high levels of economic growth since the end of the armed conflict on April 4, 2002. Its economy is essentially dependent on the oil sector, which accounts for 55% of GDP and 95% of exports. The rural sector, which includes agriculture, forestry and livestock, is the country's second largest productive sector, whose GDP is currently around 8%. According to the Human Development Index (HDI), the country ranks 160th out of 173 countries (UNDP, 2006). Despite economic growth, the majority of the Angolan population (62.2%) continues to live below the poverty line, of which 26% are in extreme poverty. The population's poverty level is reflected in poor access to food, drinking water, sanitation, education, health, electricity and other aspects (MPA, 2007). The dependency ratio is estimated at 92.3 per 100 people of working age between 15 and 64, which reflects the high unemployment rate. Despite an annual growth rate of 26% in 2006, due to the recovery of agricultural production with the return of displaced people to their places of origin, the HDI remains low, with a per capita income of USD 510 in 2002 and USD 1,980 in 2006 (WORLD BANK, 2008).

1.2.2 - **Health indicators of socio-economic interest**

The civil war that ravaged the country for 27 years, in addition to claiming human lives, displaced a third of the population from their places of origin (PEACE PLEDGE UNION, 2004), leading to the migration of a significant portion of the population with an overload of large urban centers and, consequently, a shortage of jobs, housing, educational and health institutions. The water and energy supply is degraded and insufficient, basic sanitation is precarious and there is a growth in the informal economy; this situation is conditioned, at least in part, by the government's priority of defending the country.

The state of health of the Angolan population is characterized by a low life expectancy at birth of around 46 years. The epidemiological picture has been dominated by communicable diseases such as malaria (the main cause of death), acute diarrheal diseases, acute respiratory diseases, tuberculosis, trypanosomiasis, immunopreventable diseases such as measles and tetanus, among others. The results of the latest HIV seroprevalence surveys indicate prevalence rates below 5% (MINISTRY OF HEALTH OF ANGOLA, 2009; WHO 2009), considered low in relation to the average for countries in the southern region, due to the armed conflict which limited the movement of people from their respective areas of residence (MINISTRY OF HEALTH OF ANGOLA, 2010). Although the overall HIV prevalence rate in Angola is around 5%, studies carried out in some regions of the country show a prevalence of 75% of cases in the 15 to 45 age group (INLS, 2006). With regard to other diseases, malaria, tuberculosis and acute diarrheal diseases are among the causes of the high infant mortality rate, which is considered to be the second highest infant mortality rate (260/1000 live births) in the world, while the fertility rate is 6.7 children per woman (M P A, 2003; MPA, 2007).

From 1975 to 1992, the Angolan National Health System was based exclusively on the principles of universal and free primary health care. From 1992, with the approval of the SNS Basic Law No. 21-B/92, the Angolan state ceased to have exclusivity and introduced user participation, with the payment of a moderating fee for the provision of health services. Health care is currently provided by the public and private sectors and is briefly structured into two main areas: public health and hospital care. The public health area is responsible for programs aimed at the major endemic diseases, namely malaria, trypanosomiasis, tuberculosis and AIDS, as well as programs aimed at health promotion and disease prevention, including maternal health, child health and an expanded vaccination program. The health care delivery system is subdivided into three hierarchical levels.

The first level or primary health care, represented by health posts, health centers, municipal hospitals, nursing posts and doctors' offices, is the first point of contact the population has with the health system. The secondary or intermediate level, represented by provincial and general hospitals, is the reference level for the first level units. The tertiary or national level, represented by differentiated and specialized hospitals, is the reference level for secondary level health units. Health care is provided by the public, private and traditional medicine sectors. In terms of infrastructure, the healthcare network consists of 1,721 health facilities, of which: eight are central hospitals; 32 provincial hospitals, 228 municipal hospitals and 1,453 health posts. At the moment, Angola has 995 Angolan doctors and 1,273 foreign doctors, making a total of 2,268 doctors.

1.2.3 - Angola's geographical and demographic situation

The Republic of Angola is located in the southern region of sub-Saharan Africa, has an area of 1,246,700 km2 and a coastline of 1,600 km from north to south. From a political-administrative point of view, the country has a presidential political regime and is divided into 18 Provinces, 164 Municipalities and 532 Communes and is in the process of political-administrative decentralization, with Luanda as the country's capital. The population density is approximately 13.2 inhabitants per km2. The Angolan population is mostly young and is estimated at 16,500,000 inhabitants (INE, 2009). Around 46.4% of the population is under 15 years of age, and the average population growth rate is 3.1% per year. Life expectancy at birth is 46 years, the infant mortality rate is 150 per thousand live births and the child mortality rate is 250 per thousand live births.

1.2.4 - Cultural and behavioral aspects of the Angolan population

Despite the scant records of Angolan culture, it is clear that women's sexuality in Angola, as in many other African regions, is not dissociated from the constitution of the family as a social entity that organizes sexual relations between the sexes. However, social control acts directly on women's bodies, identifying them as mothers and reproducers of legitimate children, giving husbands legal rights over their wives. In this dynamic, important African studies mention that men and women act in a cultural environment that establishes gender relations, habits, customs and behaviors marked by inequalities (DEGREGORI, et al., 2007), with men being the main decision-makers in the context of conjugal relationships (DEGREGORI, et al., 2007). Thus, heterosexual relations, considered to be a natural phenomenon with an instinctive basis, i.e. biologically given, are often subject to repression (CAPLAN, 1987), placing women before a peculiar phenomenon consisting of prohibitions, punishments, permissions and rewards concerning something that would be purely natural" (CHAUÍ, MARILENA 1984). This makes women's existence difficult and repressive, as lack of self-expression, economic subordinacy and domestic violence are major barriers to sexual and reproductive freedom (DUFFY, 2005). Today, women's sexuality has been influenced by the globalization of HIV/AIDS, placing them in a situation of extreme vulnerability.

Since vulnerability to HIV is a multidimensional concept, its causes are a multiple combination of different factors. Individual behaviors and attitudes can often express the social, geographical and cultural context in which they develop (DEGREGORI, et al., 2007; LOFORTE, 2007). Cultural factors are dynamic and also determine family and individual structure and behavior. For this reason, men and women act in a cultural environment that establishes gender relations, habits, customs and behaviors marked by inequalities (DEGREGORI, et al., 2007). Angola, like other African regions, has cultural peculiarities that can modify behavior and consequently increase female vulnerability to HIV. These behaviors include polygamy, gender inequality, early marriage, sexual repression and domestic violence, among others.

Early marriage

In the light of culture, certain norms can influence young people to marry as early as possible, have many children and, because of their power to face life, acquire approval, recognition and consecration at an early age (UNDP, 2001). Their biological ability to have children is culturally interpreted as a symbol of femininity (LAMPHERE, 1974; ORTNER, ROSALDO, 1976 - the main goal in life and a deviant behavior when compared to childless or sterile women. For this reason, the decision to limit fertility is contradicted by the protagonism of motherhood and the desire to perpetuate the family by bearing a child, regardless of any inherent risk to life and, consequently, contributing to high fertility, birth and maternal mortality rates (INE, 2003), among other indicators.

Gender inequality and sexual repression

Culturally defined values in the community based on gender limit the ability to make choices about sexual and reproductive health, thus making sexuality "taboo". African studies show that men are primarily responsible for deciding the context of family relationships, contraceptive use and family size, and that communication and discussions between spouses about health, family and family planning are scarce, thus disregarding any desire on the part of women to control their bodies, reduce the number of children or delay births (DEGREGORI, et al., 2007). Resistance to the use of contraceptives, linked to the desire to have children induced by previously assumed cultural, economic and emotional imperatives, and the lack of information about sexual and reproductive health are classic examples. Often, the presence of illnesses related to sexual behavior represents a concern beyond family responsibilities: those involved feel more free to confide in their families (AGADJANIAN, 2001). Many young people say that little information about sex is obtained mainly from friends and people of a relatively older age, as the intention to discuss sex with older people is considered disrespectful (DEGREGORI, et al., 2007).

Sex education in African culture takes different forms. Some parents, considered to be conservative, appoint a family member (aunt) to be responsible for sexual education in relation to the start of a relationship, traditional formalities for consensual unions, obligations and marital duties of young women (GARCIA, 1995). Another form of education consists of leaving the mother in charge of teaching about female sexuality, where aspects concerning marital duties and obligations, domestic care and others are covered (JUNIOR, 1995). However, others, although they no longer value sexual education in the light of African culture because they consider themselves modern, maintain, like the others, the image of women as objects of desire, socially legitimizing them as dependent on men without the right to negotiate a protected sexual relationship, above all, dissociating themselves from genuine polygamy (DEGREGORI, et al., 2007) (understood as a conjugal relationship between a man and a defined number of - more than two - female partners, giving them all the status of wife, assuming the role of provider and the commitment to fidelity, among other obligations, without, however, the coexistence of relationships with another partner outside this circuit).

Gender relations

A more detailed analysis of gender-related factors in sub-Saharan Africa shows that the biological, cultural, economic and social status of women can increase the likelihood of HIV infection (DELAY, 2004; KALIPENI, et al., 2007). Some cultural beliefs and practices foster and maintain gender inequalities at the top of women's vulnerability to HIV. In Zimbabwe, DUFFY (2005) demonstrated that women's existence is difficult and oppressed, and observed that lack of freedom of expression, economic subordination and domestic violence constitute important barriers to HIV prevention. From a socio-cultural point of view, women are more affected and conditioned by the different statuses in the family structure that they have assumed in the different stages of the life cycle. Her authority, autonomy, responsibility, obligations and occupation change according to the variations between being a daughter, mother, daughter-in-law, mother-in-law, married, widowed or single (LOFORTE, 2007).

Polygamy

African studies (KALIPENI, et al., 2007) point to cultural peculiarities that figure as influential behavioral factors in the growing HIV/AIDS epidemic. Some scholars point to peculiar aspects of sexuality such as polygamy, the inheritance of widows and the sexual violation of virgin girls, among others, which characterize the behaviour of African men (RUSHING, 1995; SHANNON et al., 1991; OPPONG and KALIPENI, 1999). In this paradigm, the existence of multiple sexual partnerships is more socially acceptable than in other cultures and has been practiced in the form of polygamy, leaving women unable to control their sex lives (MACDONALD, 1996). However, this behavior does not translate into extramarital sexual relations involving other women. Traditional African polygamy is defined as the act of maintaining a marriage, i.e. a conjugal relationship with more than one partner, all of whom maintain the status of wife, while the man assumes the commitment of fidelity and provider, among other obligations. This situation keeps women submissive and inferior, excluded from decision-making power, exposed to domestic violence, lack of sexual and reproductive freedom, changing their daily behavior as well as their perception of the risk of becoming infected with HIV, (SILVA, e VARGENS, 2009; BUCHALLA e PAIVA., 2002; SALDANHA, 2005;

WERNECK, 2005). Nevertheless, some studies have shown an inverse relationship between HIV/AIDS rates and polygamy rates (KALIPENI, ET AL 1998; GHOSH, J, AWIRE-VALHMU, L M, 2007). In North Africa, where polygamy is more frequent and strongly rooted in Islamic societies, HIV/AIDS rates have been shown to be the lowest in the whole continent (TASTEMAIN and COLES 1993; KALIPENI and OPPONG, 1998). This may explain the high HIV/AIDS rates among the younger population, supposedly because they are dissociated from the traditional polygamy mentioned above.

Domestic violence

According to the WHO, domestic violence is defined as violence perpetuated by very close people within family relationships, including intimate partners, and can be of a psychological, physical or sexual nature. Its domestic nature often means that it is no longer understood as violence by society (SCHRAIBER, et al, 2005); this is also true in Angolan/African culture, where family, individual and gender contexts represent the main foundations of its occurrence (STARK and FLITCRAFT, 1991).

Studying domestic violence from a sociocultural perspective (GARCIA-MORENO et al., 2007; (SCHRAIBERI et al., 2010 as a theoretical basis for vulnerability to HIV in the Angolan female population seems to be extremely valuable, since violence is a relevant factor for various health outcomes (CAMPBELL , 2002; ELLSBERG et al...), 2008; JEWKES et al. 2002; KRUG et al., 2002), above all because it occurs in asymmetrical and hierarchical interpersonal relationships (RAVAZZOLA, 1997, 1999; WHO, REDESAÚDE, 2001; CORSI, 1997, 2003) already referred to in the light of the prevailing culture, (SCHRAIBER et al., 2010; (GARCIA-MORENO et al., 2005; GARCIA-MORENO et al., 2003; SCHRAIBER et al., 2007;). Some studies on violent behavior (DAHLBERG & KRUG, 2003; HEISE & GARCIA-MORENO et al., 2003) associate the practice of violent acts with beliefs and cultural backgrounds, without therefore considering it as the practice of violence. In this way, associated cultural peculiarities such as polygamy and gender inequality, among others, can influence the occurrence of violence to a certain extent, conditioning a situation of vulnerability.

This study focuses on the gender perspective in Angolan culture, understanding violence as a product of conflicts in heterosexual relationships that can lead to female vulnerability to HIV.

1.2.5 - Characterization of the study site

The Augusto Ngangula Maternity Hospital (MAG), where the study was carried out, is located in Luanda, capital of Angola, and is a national reference center for high-risk prenatal care by the Ministry of Health (MS). It is also accredited for teaching activities at postgraduate level by the Ministry of Health (MoH) and the Agostinho Neto University (UAN). It offers gynecology, obstetrics and neonatology services, laboratory and radiological diagnostic support services, a 24-hour emergency service and outpatient services in a wide range of subspecialties. Due to the growing number of HIV cases in the country, a service for pregnant women with HIV/AIDS was set up as a strategic measure to control vertical transmission. According to the information available at the time of collecting the data for this study, the prenatal care service sees 15 to 20 pregnant women a day, either by referral or on demand.

Chapter 2

2- OBJECTIVES
2.1 - General
To estimate the frequency of risk factors for sexual transmission of HIV in HIV-positive pregnant women and HIV-negative pregnant women using the public health network in Luanda, Angola, and to verify their association with HIV/AIDS infection, during the period from August 2007 to December 2009.
2.2 - Specifics
2.2.1   To estimate the frequency of potential risk factors for sexual transmission of HIV in HIV-positive and HIV-negative pregnant women

2.2.2   To verify the association between HIV/AIDS infection and potential risk factors for sexual transmission of HIV:

Socio-economic factors: education, occupation, personal income/head of household, personal expenses, inhabited (type of dwelling), energy, water, household goods

Demographic factors: age, marital status, household, place of birth, residence, ethnicity

Political factors: coming from a war zone, migration, imprisonment or military captivity, military service

Cultural factors: previous marital union, initiative in the relationship, religion, partner's age, polygamy, temporary separation, controlling behavior by the partner, psychological, physical, sexual, physical violence by another family member

Characteristics and behavior of the women studied: partner's serology, number of previous sexual partners, condom use with a steady partner, condom use with an occasional partner, sex under the influence of alcohol (start of sexual activity, contraceptive used, presence of STDs.

Characteristics and behavior of the partners of the women studied: Age, schooling, length of time living with partner, frequenting barbershops, use of alcoholic beverages.

<h1 style="text-align:center">Chapter 3</h1>

3- METHODOLOGY

3.1 - Design and study population

This was a hospital-based case-control study involving 1092 pregnant women, 273 of whom tested positive for HIV - considered to be **cases,** and 819 of whom tested negative for HIV - considered to be **controls,** selected during prenatal consultations at the Augusto Ngangula maternity hospital in Luanda - Angola, over a period of 28 (twenty-eight) months, from August 2007 to November 2009. The study population was made up of pregnant women who spontaneously sought the service as well as those who were referred for specific follow-up at the high-risk prenatal clinic.

3.2 - Procedures for selecting study groups

The patients were selected at the antenatal clinic after pre-test counseling and a rapid HIV test. After the test result, all the pregnant women were called in for a chat to inform them about the study and invite them to take part. Those who agreed were taken to the interview room where, after the objectives of the research had been explained in detail, the consent form was signed and the questionnaire was administered. Those pregnant women who tested positive for HIV (rapid test) became cases. Pregnant women who had a negative HIV rapid test were selected as controls until the estimated sample size was reached, maintaining the ratio of 3 controls for each case. Women with dubious serological test results were excluded from the study.

3.3 - Sample calculation

The sample size of the study population was calculated based on the following parameters: alpha error of 5%, beta error of 20%, study power of 80% and a difference in frequencies (54/44) between cases and controls for the education variable. In this variable, the category "low schooling" was considered from a total of 100 women who allowed the previous pilot study to be carried out, and yet one case for 3 controls was estimated, with 273 cases and 819 controls totaling 1092 cases, the sample for the present study.

3.4 - Analysis variables

Definition of study groups (dependent variable)

HIV-positive women were considered cases, as were patients who showed serological evidence of HIV by reacting to the rapid test <u>(VIKIA HIV 1/2 from bio Merieux)</u> and controls were patients who, after undergoing the rapid HIV test, showed negative serological evidence of HIV.

Dependent variable/independent variables

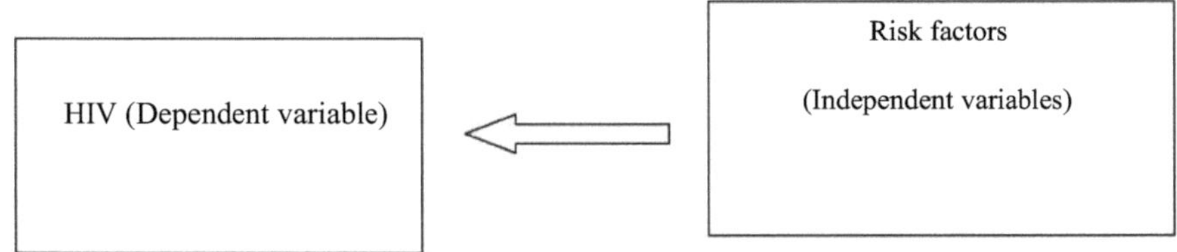

3.5 - Conceptual model

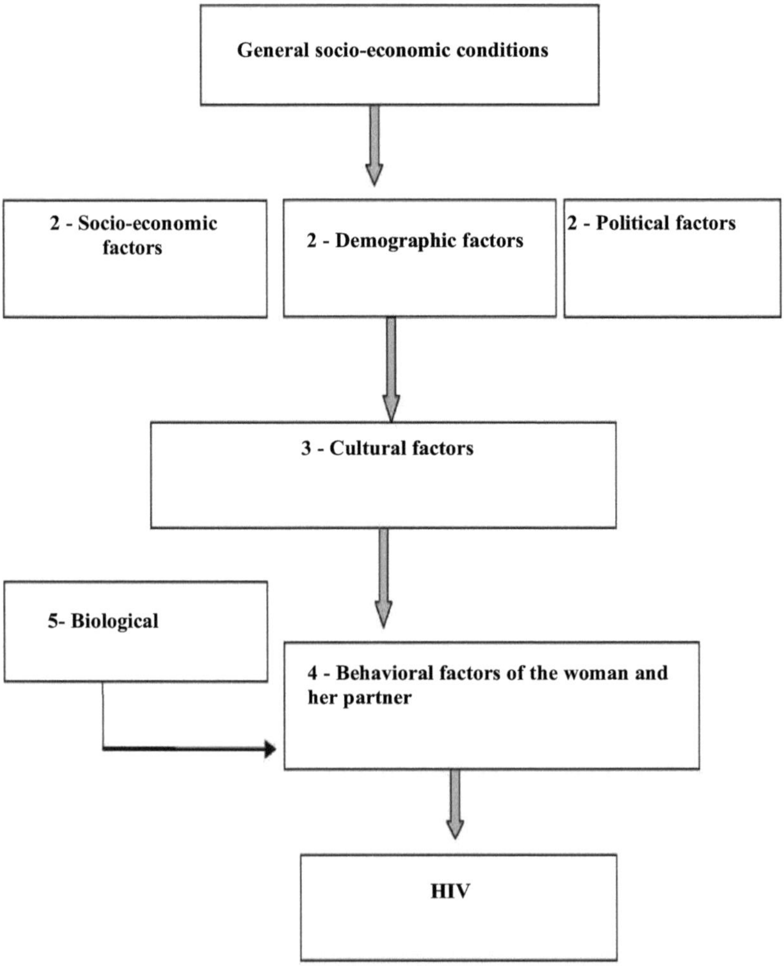

Figure 1 - Conceptual model for sexual transmission of HIV in women

3.6 - Operational definitions for terms and variables

The risk factors for sexual transmission of HIV (demographic, socioeconomic, political, cultural and behavioral) were grouped by blocks of variables, according to a previously established conceptual model comprising different levels of determination (Figure 1).

According to the diagram above, general socioeconomic and demographic factors represent level 1 (distal); demographic, socioeconomic and political factors represent level 2 (intermediate); cultural factors represent level 3 (intermediate); behavioral factors represent level 4 (intermediate); biological factors represent level 5 (proximal).

3.6.1 - Demographic variables

Demographic variables were taken into account: age, marital status, nationality, place of birth, family situation, family agglomeration, residence and ethnicity.

Age - continuous numerical variable expressed in years, counted from the date of birth to the moment of hospital admission for participation in the study and must be in accordance with the individual's identity record presented at the consultation. categorization: up to 29 years old, from 30 to 49 years old.

Marital status: marital status is the condition in which a woman finds herself in relation to marriage or marital status according to the Brazilian Constitution (Law 9.278/96). - polytomous nominal categorical variable. Categories: single (those who have never married, or who have had their marriage annulled), married (those who have entered into marriage, regardless of the property regime adopted).

Household - refers to the number of individuals, regardless of age, living in the household and sharing a table. Categories: up to 3 people, 4 to 6 people, 7 and over.

Place of birth: referred to as the place where the woman interviewed was born Categories:

Luanda, other provinces, abroad.

Residence: refers to the administrative area of habitual residence corresponding to the neighborhood and municipality of Luanda where you currently live. Polychotomous nominal variable. Categories: RLM, other municipalities, other province.

Ethnicity: defined according to the national language spoken, bringing up the "Bantu" ethnic origin Categories: kimbundo, umbundo, kicongo, other, foreign

3.6.2 - Socio-economic variables

1 - Socio-economic risk factors according to the productive insertion of the woman and the head of household

Schooling: Schooling - refers to the number of years of schooling completed by the woman: polychotomous nominal variable. Categories: illiterate, primary education, secondary education, higher education

Occupation: - refers to the type of activity carried out by the woman. It was categorized as: public servant, self-employed, housewife, student

Personal income: 150 USD was chosen as the cut-off point because it is the minimum wage currently in force in Angola. Categories: no income, don't know, up to 300 dollars, over 300 dollars

Income of the head of household: 150 USD was chosen as the cut-off point because it is the minimum wage currently in force in Angola. Categories: no income, up to 300 dollars, over 300 dollars

Personal expenses: personal expenses were considered to be the amount in dollars corresponding to what the woman spends per month on individual needs, i.e,
items or products that you don't share with other family members. Categories: under 150 dollars, 150 to 300 dollars, over 300 dollars

Type of dwelling - qualitatively classifies the type of dwelling where the research subject lives, taking into account the material used in its construction. Polychotomous nominal categorical variable. Categories: masonry, other

Water supply: refers to the origin of the water supply used for domestic consumption such as hygiene and food preparation. Polychotomous nominal categorical variable. Categories: piped water, fountain, cistern supply

Electricity supply: refers to the consumption of electricity as well as another source if there is no public supply network. Categories: with power, generator supply, without power

Ownership of household goods: refers to the use of household consumer goods. Categories: one good, two to four goods, five to six goods

3.6.3 - Political variables

Military mobilization: women who declared themselves to be in the armed forces or any other branch of the military in full exercise were considered to be mobilized Polytomous nominal categorical variable. Categories: not mobilized, mobilized

Critical background to the war (war situations): refers to the story referred to by the woman portraying a critical life under the effects of the rekindling of the civil war in Angola. Polychotomous nominal categorical variable. Categories: did not experience situations, experienced situations

3.6.4 - Cultural variables

Previous marital union. Refers to the woman's previous marital history before the current union. Categories : one union, two or more unions

Relationship initiative: refers to the person who takes the initiative to start a marital/love relationship. categories: man, woman

Religion: refers to the name of the religious belief that the woman professes. Categories : with religion, without religion

Age of partner: the woman declared the age of her partner in complete years. Categories: 20 to 29 years; 30 to 39 years, 40 years and over, unknown

Polygamy: refers to a man's marital relationship with a defined number of partners (more than two), all of whom have the status of wife, assuming the role of provider and the commitment of fidelity, among other obligations, without, however, the coexistence of relationships with another partner outside this circuit). categories: no other wife, has another wife, 2 to 4 wives, five wives and more

Temporary separation: refers to the possibility of having been separated for some time during your relationship with your current partner. Categories: never, yes

Controlling partner behavior: a form of violence practiced by an intimate partner that characterizes some kind of aggressive and abusive behavior. Categories:
1- You fight; 2- Prevents you from visiting friends/neighbors; 3- Tries to restrict your contact with family; 4- Has tended to your concerns or feelings; 5- Insists on knowing where you are at all times; 6- Ignores you and treats you with indifference; 7- Gets

angry if you talk to another man; 8- Is often suspicious of you; 9- Is always suspicious of you before seeking care for his own health. Suspecting you of being unfaithful; 9- Always waits for you to get permission before seeking care for his own health; 10- None of the above has occurred; 88- not applicable; 99- no information. **For analysis, the data was recategorized into yes (those who declared that they had experienced any of the categories mentioned) and no (when no category was declared).**

Psychological violence: a form of violence practiced by an intimate partner that characterizes some kind of aggressive behavior of a psychological nature. Categories: 1- Insults and makes you feel bad about yourself ; 2- Depressed or humiliated you in front of other people; 3- Did things to scare you or frighten you on purpose (shouted, broke things, etc.); 4- Threatened to hurt you or someone you care about; 5- none of these situations occurred; 88 - not applicable; 99- no information. **For analysis, they were recategorized into yes (those who declared that they had experienced any of the categories mentioned) and no (when no category was declared).**

Physical violence: form of violence practiced by an intimate partner that characterizes some kind of aggressive behavior of a physical nature. Categories: 1- He got angry enough to hit you (slap, punch, shove, kick, beat); 2- Has he assaulted you with a gun or knife?3 - Has he ever assaulted you during pregnancy; 4 - Has he ever tried to strangle you on purpose; 5 - Has he ever promised to kill you; 6 - Has he ever needed medical attention to treat injuries caused by physical assault; 7 - Have you ever reported any of the assaults you have suffered to the police; 8 - Have you ever reported any of the assaults you have suffered to your family, church, OMA; 9 - Has he ever tried to burn you on purpose; 10 - None of the above; 88 - Not applicable; 99 - No information. **For analysis, it was recategorized into yes (those who declared having experienced any of the categories mentioned) and no (when no category was declared).**

Sexual violence is a form of interpersonal violence committed by an intimate partner or family member against a woman in a superior position (physical, age, social, psychological and/or hierarchical) characterized by coercive behaviour that forces a woman to have sex in order to violate her autonomy, physical or psychological integrity. Categories: 1- he physically forced you to have sex when you didn't want to; 2- you had to do it because you were afraid of his reaction; 3- he forced you into a degrading or humiliating sexual practice; 10- none of these situations occurred 88 - not applicable; 99- no information. **For the purposes of analysis, they were recategorized into yes (those who declared that they had experienced any of the categories mentioned) and no (when no category was declared).**

3.6.5 - Behavioral variables

1 - women's sexual behavior

The following behavioral variables were considered for the women: partner's serology, number of previous sexual partners, condom use with a steady partner, condom use with an occasional partner, sex under the influence of alcohol.

Partner's HIV status: did the woman say she knew or didn't know about HIV? Categories: HIV+, HIV-, don't know

Number of partners: refers to the number of sexual partners a woman has had during her sexual life. Categories: one partner, two partners, three partners, four and more

Reason for not using condoms with a steady partner. categories: married, using another method, careless, he doesn't like it
Condom use with occasional partner. categories: no occasional partner, no use, use
Sexual intercourse under the influence of alcohol: refers to sexual intercourse under the influence of alcohol. Categories: yes, no

2 - Partner characteristics and behavior

The following behavioral variables of the partners were considered: age, schooling, length of time living with partner, frequency of barbering, use of alcoholic beverages. Polychotomous variables.

Partner's age - continuous numerical variable expressed in years, counted from the date of birth to the moment of hospital admission for participation in the study and must be in accordance with the individual's identity record presented at the consultation. categorization:

20 to 29 years old, 30 to 39 years old, over 49 years old, don't know

Using a barber for a haircut: yes, no

Alcohol consumption: refers to the habit of drinking alcoholic beverages: categories: yes, no

Schooling: Schooling - refers to the number of years of schooling completed by the woman: polychotomous nominal variable. Categories: primary education, secondary education, higher education and more, unknown

Length of time living with partner: refers to the length of time, defined in years, that the woman has been living with her sexual partner. Categories: less than 1 year, one to five years, more than five years, unknown

3.7 - Data collection and storage

Data was collected in two stages. Initially, a pilot study involving 50 cases and 50 controls was carried out in order to gather data that would serve as a basis for calculating the sample size, and to test the clarity and effectiveness of the questionnaire. After analyzing the pilot, some questions could be reformulated and others eliminated, which culminated in the preparation of the definitive questionnaire, which was applied to the study population to answer the proposed objectives.

3.8 - Data processing and analysis

The data was stored in a database in the statistical program EPI-INFO 6.04 b (CDC, Atlanta, USA), with double entry of data and the use of the *"validate"* program to check and correct any typing errors. The data collected allowed for the construction of a database in the EPI-INFO statistical program, which was analyzed using the STATA 8.2 statistical package (Copyright 1984-2003). For analysis, the variables were grouped into blocks. Initially, a univariate analysis was carried out, checking the association of each variable with HIV infection. The Odds Ratio was calculated with the respective 95% confidence intervals and the "p" value. Variables with a p-value < 0.20 in the association with the outcome were entered into an intra-block multivariate model. Those variables with a p-value of <0.05 remained in the final model.

3.9 - Methodological limitations

The type of study design adopted makes it susceptible to bias, particularly because the outcome and exposure have already occurred.

(RODRIGUES AND WERNECK, 2003). The main methodological limitations of this study and the strategies adopted to minimize them will be discussed below.

According to Medronho (2003), the selection of cases in case-control studies requires a clear and standardized definition of the outcome of interest, as well as a clear choice of incident or prevalent cases. In this study we chose to include pregnant women attending prenatal care after testing for HIV seropositivity using the rapid test. As cases and controls were selected from the same antenatal clinic, they came from the same population of origin and were therefore comparable in terms of geographical area of residence, socio-economic and political conditions, and cultural background.

Selecting only pregnant women limits the possibility of extrapolating the results to other groups of non-pregnant women. On the other hand, studies that take pregnant women as a reference are particularly relevant, due to the fact that they make up a significant proportion of women of reproductive age and with an active sex life, and due to the potential impact of interventions on the health of these women and on sexual and vertical transmission. It should be noted, however, that the results obtained in this study cannot be automatically extrapolated to pregnant women who do not receive prenatal care.

Incident cases represent new cases that arise, while prevalent cases represent individuals with the disease (event) in a given period of time. The selection of prevalent cases allows a greater number of subjects to be included, but the long duration of the disease can lead to a change in habits or exposure conditioned by the time elapsed since the diagnosis was made. In this study, the cases selected were newly diagnosed (minutes before the interview), so there was no time for knowledge of the infection to influence the patients' habits.

With regard to information and recall biases, questions about aspects of personal and emotional life may have caused concern and, consequently, distortion in the recall and information of several of the latents surveyed. This problem could be exacerbated if knowledge of serological status influences the ability to recall the information requested. To minimize these biases, a questionnaire with closed questions and simple, clear language was designed and administered by the same interviewer. In addition, patients were approached in a private setting, with guarantees of confidentiality and anonymity, and educational material was offered after the consultation.

The possibility of misclassification in the diagnosis of HIV infection cannot be ruled out. However, as the rapid test used (VIKIA HIV 1/2 from bioMerieux) has a sensitivity and specificity of approximately 99%, according to the manufacturer's information, the error is small and would be a non-differential misclassification.

ETHICAL CONSIDERATIONS

This study complied with the ethical guidelines for research involving human beings (World Medical Association, 2002); Brazil, Ministry of Health, 1996). It was submitted to and approved by the Ethics Committees of the National Institute for the Fight against AIDS, the Augusto Ngangula Hospital in Luanda and UFPE before data collection began. Free and informed written consent was requested from the patients, ensuring the confidentiality and exclusivity of the data for scientific purposes.

Chapter 4
RESULTS

After processing and analyzing the data, the results were generated and will be presented in the form of articles:

ARTICLE 1* - Association between demographic, socio-economic and political factors and sexual transmission of HIV in pregnant women

ARTICLE 2* - Association between cultural factors and sexual transmission of HIV in pregnant women

ARTICLE 3* - Association between behavioral factors and sexual transmission of HIV in pregnant women

ARTICLE 1* - Association between demographic, socio-economic and political factors and sexual transmission of HIV in pregnant women

Association between demographic, socio-economic and political factors and sexual transmission of HIV in pregnant women

ABSTRACT: **Introduction:** Studies on the determinants of HIV infection in African women are scarce in the literature. **Objectives: To** identify demographic, socioeconomic and political factors associated with HIV infection in Angolan women. **Method: A** case-control study involving 1092 pregnant women, of whom 273 were cases (women with positive HIV serology) and 819 were controls (women with negative HIV serology), selected from prenatal care at the Augusto Ngangula maternity hospital in Luanda, Angola, between 2007 and 2009. **Results:** Of the 1092 pregnant women, 63.1% belonged to the 30-49 age group, 94.7% were married and 54.8% were from Luanda. The majority belonged to the Quimbundo ethnic group (66.0%) and 2.4% had experienced war. The following factors showed an independent association with HIV infection: Demographic: age, place of residence and ethnicity; Socio-economic: occupation, personal and head of household income, type of housing, water and energy supply and ownership of household goods; Political: having experienced war situations **Conclusions:** The association of HIV with age suggests an increased prevalence of infection from the age of 30 and consequently a probable under-reporting in younger women, implying women's health policies aimed at this group and encouraging voluntary serological testing for HIV before pregnancy. Socio-economic status showed no clear association with HIV infection, suggesting a double pattern, thus highlighting the complexity of the network of determinants of infection.

Key Words : HIV, sexual transmission, pregnant women, risk factors

Association between demographic, socioeconomic and political factors and HIV infection in pregnant women

SUMMARY: **Background**: Studies on the determinants of HIV infection in African women are scarce in the literature. **Objectives:** To identify demographic, socioeconomic and political factors associated with HIV infection in Angolan women. **Methods:** A case control study was conducted, comprising 1092 pregnant women of which 273 were cases (women who were seropositive) and 819 were controls (women who were seronegative), selected from the antenatal maternity Ngangula of Luanda-Angola in the period 2007 to 2009. **Results:** Of the 1092 pregnant women, 63.1% were aged 30 to 49 years, 94.7% were married, and 54.8% were born in Luanda. Most of them belonged to the Quimbundo ethnicity (66.0%)and 2.4% experienced situations of war. The following factors were independently associated with HIV infection: Demographic: age, place of residence and ethnicity; Socioecnomic: occupation, personal income and income of the head of the family, housing, water supply, energy and possession of goods; Political: having experienced war situations. **CONCLUSIONS:** The association of HIV with age suggests an increased prevalence of infection from 30 years and therefore a likely underreporting in younger women, highlighting the importance of developing health policies targeting this group and the need to encourage HIV serologic testing before pregnancy. The socioeconomic status showed no clear association with HIV infection suggesting a double pattern, thus underlining the complexity of the network of the determinants of infection.

Keywords: HIV, sexual transmission, pregnant women, risk factors

INTRODUCTION

HIV infection has gone from a simple case report to a worldwide epidemic, leading to significant repercussions from a socio-economic, anthropological, political and cultural point of view, among others (GALVÄO, et al 2000). According to global estimates, the number of people living with HIV in the world increased from 29.0 to 33.4 million between 2001 and 2008, and 2.0 million deaths occurred in 2008. In this scenario, sub-Saharan Africa is the region most affected, contributing 67% of all infections and 72% of all deaths (UNAIDS & WHO, 2009). Studies on the epidemiological profile of HIV in the world have revealed a heterosexual character and feminization, as well as the impoverishment and internalization of HIV (BRITO et al 2000; NETO, J.F.R et al, 2010) with notable regional variations, especially in the poorest countries such as those on the African continent (CASTILHO and CHEQUER, 1997; CASTILHO et al...), 1999; OLINTO and GALVÄO, 1999; UNAIDS, 2004; PARKER, 2000; NETO, 2010). As early as the 1980s, the proportion of women with HIV was significant, even in developed countries such as the United States and the United Kingdom, reaching 20% in Europe compared to 50% in Africa (JONES, 1989).

According to UNAIDS statistics (2009), of the total of 31.3 million adults living with HIV, 15.7 million represent the global female population. In sub-Saharan Africa, out of a total of 22.4 million people living with HIV, 60% are women, with Botswana (25.0%), South Africa (16.9%) and Zambia (14.6%) being the countries with the highest prevalence in this population. A study involving pregnant women in Angolan border regions showed a low seroprevalence (2.8%) (INLS, 2005), compared to 37% in Botswana and 21.0% in Zambia, also observed in pregnant women.

Vulnerability to HIV was initially identified in large urban centers, where homosexuals, injecting drug users and recipients of blood and blood products represented the main risk groups. Subsequent studies found that in addition to the factors listed above, other socioeconomic, demographic, political, cultural and behavioral aspects made up the vulnerability to infection. With regard to female vulnerability and particularly in sub-Saharan Africa, in addition to biological susceptibility in heterosexual relationships and other factors mentioned, polygamy, violence and inequalities in gender relations are among the diversity of risk factors for HIV transmission (SEFFNER, 1998; UNAIDS, 2009; KHOBOTLO et al., 2009;

ANDERSSON et al., 2007).

In Angola, the political, demographic, cultural and socio-economic aspects are peculiar and can make women more vulnerable to STD/AIDS, thus contributing to the high and growing rates of HIV in sub-Saharan Africa, of which Angola is a part (WHO, 1999; ANGOLA, 2001; MONTAGNIER, 1995).

With this in mind, this study aims to identify risk factors for sexual transmission of HIV in Angolan women, in order to support proposals for interventions in their sexual and reproductive health care. Studies looking at pregnant women are particularly relevant because they make up a significant proportion of women of reproductive age with an active sex life and because of the potential impact of interventions on their health and on sexual and vertical transmission.

METHODS

This is a case-control study involving 1,092 pregnant women, of whom 273 are cases and 819 are controls, selected during prenatal consultations at the Augusto Ngangula maternity hospital in Luanda, Angola, between 2007 and 2009. This institution is a national reference for the Ministry of Health and Agostinho Neto University for medical care including vertical transmission of HIV/AIDS in pregnant women and postgraduate teaching activities. Cases were women who tested positive for HIV when submitted to the rapid test and controls were women who tested negative for HIV. All ethical requirements were met, as well as submission to and approval by the ethics committees for research involving human beings at UFPE - Brazil and MINSA - Angola. The data collection technique was an individual interview, carried out in a private environment, using a semi-structured questionnaire made up of closed questions, applied by the main researcher after a pilot study which helped to estimate the population and adapt the instrument. The data collected allowed a database to be built using the EPI-INFO statistical program and analyzed using the STATA 8.2 statistical package (Copyright 19842003). The variables were initially grouped into blocks. The univariate analysis verified the association of each variable with HIV infection. Odds ratios, 95% confidence intervals and p-values were calculated. Variables with a p-value < 0.20 in the association with the outcome were included in an intra-block multivariate model. Those with a p-value < 0.010 in the intra-block model were entered into a final multivariate model. Variables with a p-value of <0.05 remained in the final model.

RESULTS

The sample was made up mainly of married women (94.7%) aged between 30 and 49 (63.1%); between 20 and 29 (34.6%), from Luanda (54.8%) and belonging to the Quimbundo ethnic group (66.0%).

Demographic risk factors

In the univariate analysis, marital status, family aggregation and place of birth were not associated with HIV infection at the 5% level. Age, place of residence and ethnicity showed an independent association with HIV infection, after intra-block adjustment and in the final model.

Table - 1 : Association between demographic risk factors (age, marital status, family aggregation) and HIV infection in pregnant women - ANG , 2007 to 2008 , Luanda-Angola

Variable	Study population		Odds	Ratio *		Odds Ratio **		
Age	Case	Control	OR	CP I		OR	IC	P
up to 29 years	58(21.25)	345(42.12)	1	-	-	-	-	-
30 a 49	215(78.8)	474(57.9)	2.70	1.96-3.72	**0.000**	3,00	2.11	- 0.000
							4.29	
State **civil**								
married	258(94.5)	776(94.7)	1	-	-	-	-	-
single	15(5.5)	43(5.3)	1.05	0.57- 1.92	0.876	-	-	-
Aggregation **family**								
up to 3 people	66 (24.2)	234 (28.6)	1	-	-	-	-	-

4a6	160(58.6)	412(50.3)	1.38	0.99-1.91	**0.056**	-	-	-
people								
7 and more	47(17.2)	173(21.1)	0.96	0.63 - 1.47	0.862	-	-	-

OR: cross product ratio; CI: confidence interval; P: P value; Gross product: unadjusted; * Odds Ratio ; ** Odds Ratio (1): adjusted for intra-block variables (marital status and family agglomeration)

Table - 2: Association between demographic risk factors (place of birth and residence) and HIV infection in pregnant women - M ANG , 2007 to 2008 , Luanda-Angola

Variable	Pop.	study	Odds Ratio *			Odds Ratio	**	
Natural	Case	Control	OR	IC	P	OR	IC	P
age								
Luanda	161	437	1	-	-			
	(59.0)	(53.4)						
Another prov	109	367	0.81	0.61-1.07	0.131	0.51	0.36-0.72	**0.000**
	(39.9)	(44.8)						
stranger	3(1.1)	15(1.8)	0.54	0.16 -1.90	**0.339**	0.12	0.02-0.72	0.020

Resid.								
RML#	26(82.8)	690(84.2)	1	-	-			
Other	36(13.2)	127(15.5)	0.87	0.58- 1.29	0.478	0.860	.56- 1.32	**0.488**
Municipa lity								
Another prov	11(4.0)	2(0.2)	16.80	3.70-6.33	**0.000**	27.04	4.56-60.50	**0.000**

OR: cross-product ratio; CI: confidence interval; P: P value; Gross product: unadjusted; * Odds Ratio ; ** Odds Ratio (1): adjusted for intra-block variables (marital status and family cluster) #RML: Luanda Metropolitan Region

Table 3: Association between demographic risk factors (ethnicity) and HIV infection in pregnant women - M ANG , 2007 to 2008 , Luanda-Angola.

Variable	Study population		Odds Ratio *			Odds Ratio **		
Ethnicity/	Case	Control	OR	IC	P	OR	IC	P
dialects								
kimbundo	165	556	1	-	-			
	(60.4)	(67.9)						

umbundo	73(26.7)	97(11.8)	2.54	1.79 - 3.60	**0.000**	3.57	2.38-5.34	**0.000**
kicongo	26(9.5)	126(15.4)	0.70	0.44 -1.10	**0.119**	0.99	0.60- 1.64	**0.602**
other	2(0.7)	29(3.5)	0.23	0.06 -0.98	**0.048**	0.16	0.02- 0.99	**0.049**
foreign	7(2.6)	11(1.3)	2.14	0.82 - 5.62	**0.121**	4.99	1.17-21.22	**0.029**

OR: cross-product ratio; CI: confidence interval; P: P value; Gross product: unadjusted; * Odds Ratio ; ** Odds Ratio (1): adjusted for intra-block variables (marital status and family cluster)

Socio-economic risk factors

The tables below show the socio-economic characteristics of the women selected in the sample. Of all the women studied (273/829), 4.6% were illiterate and (27.1%) were housewives. Approximately 73.2% of the heads of household had an income of more than 300 US dollars. Table 2 shows the socio-economic variables according to the productive insertion of the woman and the head of household, of which schooling was not associated with HIV in the univariate analysis. However, occupation, personal income and that of the head of household remained independently associated with HIV after intra-block adjustment.

Table - 4: Association between socio-economic factors according to the productive insertion of the woman and the head of household and HIV infection in pregnant women - M ANG , 2007 to 2008 , LuandaAngola

Variable	Study population		Odds Ratio *			Odds]	Ratio 1†	
Education	Case	Control	OR	IC	P	OR	IC	P
e								
illiterate	10(3.7)	38(4.6)	1	-	-	-	-	-

*** Odds Ratio ; ** Odds Ratio 1. adjusted for intra-block variables *** income of head of household D#: US Dollars**

fundamental	140(51.3)	463(56.5)	1.15	0.556-2.36	0.706	-	-	-
medium	108(39.6)	280(34.2)	1.47	0.71- 3.04	0.305	-	-	-
top	15(5.5)	38(4.6)	1.5	0.60- 3.76	0.387	-	-	-
Occupation								
F. public	74(27.1)	136(16.6)	1	-	-	-	-	-
Autonomous	93 (34.1)	307(37.5)	0.56	0.39-0 .80	0.002	0.99	0.58 - 1.40	0.640
From home	82(30.0)	222(27.1)	0.68	0.46-0 .99	0.046	1.16	0.64- 13.93	0.698
Student	24(8.8)	142(17.3)	0.31	0.19-0.52	0.000	0.44	0.24- 0.81	0.008
Income staff								
no income don't know	89(32.6) 30(11.0)	323(39.4) 169(20.6)	1 0.64	- 0.41-1.01	- 0.058	0.64	0.34 - 1.19	0.157
up to 300 D	98(35.9)	216(26,2)	1.65	1.18- 2.30	0.003	1.67	1.04-2.68	0.033
>300D	56(20,6)	111(13,5)	1.83	1.23- 2.73	0.003	1.77	1.01-3.10	0.045
Income boss								

no income up to 300 D#	12(4.4) 60(22,0)	13(1.6) 153(18,7)	1 0.42	- 0.18-0.99	- 0.046	0.35	0.14-0.81	0.017
>300D	200(73,2)	644(78,7)	0.35	0.15-0.75	0.008	0.34	0.15-0.78	0.011

OR: cross product ratio; CI: confidence interval; P: P value

In the group of socio-economic variables according to the woman's consumption pattern, only the type of housing, water supply and ownership of goods maintained an independent association with HIV in the multivariate analysis, after intra-block adjustment - table 3

Table - 4: Association between socio-economic factors according to women's consumption patterns and HIV infection in women - M ANG , 2007 to 2008 , Luanda-Angola

Variable	Study population		Odds Ratio *			Odds Ratio **1		
Expenses	Case	Control	OR	IC	P	OR	IC	P
personal								
< 150D	196(71.8)	702(85.7)	1	-	-	-	-	-
150- 300D	70(25.6)	107(13.1)	2.34	1.67- 3.29	0.000	-	-	-
> 300D	7(2.6)	10(1.2)	2.51	0.94- 6.67	0.066	-	-	-
Type inhabited masonry	264(96.7)	810(98.9)	1	-	-	-	-	-
others	9(3.3)	9(1.1)	3.07	1.21-7.81	0.019	3.01	1.09-8.33	0.033
Abast.								
water								
Network P.	104(38.1)	325(39.7)	1	-	-			

Fountain	86(31.5)	306(37.4)	0.89	0.63- 1.22	0.435	1.56	1.08-2.25	0.017
Cistern	83(30.4)	188(23.0)	1.38	0.98- 1.94	0.063	2.86	1.93-4.24	0.000
Energy								
electrical								
with	245(89.7)	621(75.8)	1	-	-			
energy								
generator	25(9.2)	104(12.7)	0.61	0.38-0.97	0.035	-	-	-
without	3(11.1)	94(11.5)	0.08	0.03-0.26	0.000	-	-	-
energy								
Assets*								
a	15(5.5)	254(31.0)	1	-	-			
2-4 goods	181 (66.31)	504 (60.74)	6.08	3.52-10.52	0.000	6.08	3.52-10.52	0.000
5- 6 goods	77(28,2)	61(7,4)	21.37	11.50-39.72	0.000	21.37	11.50-39.72	0.000

OR: cross product ratio; CI: confidence interval; P: P value * Odds Ratio ; ** Odds Ratio 1. adjusted for intra block variables ***household goods

<u>**Political risk factors**</u>

Table 4 shows the block of political variables characterized by mobilization for military service, situations experienced during the civil war.

As for mobilization, 2.9% of the women had been in the military and 5.1% had experienced war. Of the political variables evaluated, only having experienced war showed a statistically significant association with HIV in the univariate analysis, although it did not remain so in the multivariate analysis with variables from all the blocks.

Table - 6: Association between political risk factors and HIV infection in women - M ANG , 2007 to 2008 , Luanda-Angola

Variable	Study population		Odds Ratio*		
Military mobilization	Case	Control	OR	IC	P
not mobilized	265(97.1)	790(96.5)	1	-	-
mobilized	8(2.9)	29(3.5)	0.82	0.37 1.82	0.630
War situations					
has not experienced	259(94.9)	807(98.5)	1	-	-
experienced situations	14(5.1)	12(1.5)	3.64	1.66 - 7.96	**0.001**

OR: cross product ratio; CI: confidence interval; P: P value * Odds Ratio

Chapter 5

DISCUSSION OF RESULTS

The results of this study showed that socio-economic, demographic and political conditions are associated with the sexual transmission of HIV.

Demographic factors

Several studies on demographic factors have shown that they are associated with HIV (BRASIL, 2010; SHISANA, 2005; SZWARCWALD, et al,2008; MUULA, 2008). In this study, age, place of birth, residence and ethnicity were independently associated with HIV infection.

As far as age is concerned, the findings differ as to whether age is lower or higher in terms of vulnerability to HIV. It is likely that methodological issues such as the number of samples, the design adopted and the location of the study may explain these differences. In this study, women aged between 30 and 49 had a greater chance of HIV infection than younger women. This finding leads to a different interpretation. Research in several countries, including African countries in the sub-Saharan region, points to a growing epidemic among younger women (BRASIL, 2010; SHISANA, 2005; SZWARCWALD, et al,2008; MUULA, 2008; IRFF, et al, 2008).

The association between HIV and age in the present study was in agreement with other researchers (SANTOS et al., 2009), suggesting an increased prevalence of infection from the age of 30 and consequently underreporting in younger women, implying that women's health policies should target this group and encourage voluntary HIV testing before pregnancy. A cross-sectional study carried out to draw up a profile of women living with HIV/AIDS compared to women using public women's health care services whose serology was unknown showed that the proportion of women over 30 in the infected group was higher than in the comparison group (SANTOS et al., 2009).

On the other hand, other studies have identified a higher prevalence in the under-30 age group, as reported by SHISANA et al, (2009) in South Africa, who found an HIV prevalence of 32.7 in the 25-29 age group, as well as by SILVEIRA et al (2008), who identified a prevalence of 27.1 and 26.4 in the 20-24 and 25-29 age groups, respectively. These findings point to a divergence in the association between HIV and age below and/or above 30. The fact that these were prevalence studies with limitations in identifying the time of infection probably explains these results. No incidence studies were found in the literature consulted to support this discussion.

References to the internalization of HIV in Angola are scarce (INLS, 2005). The available evidence suggests an increased risk of infection in the interior in high-prevalence sub-Saharan countries (MUULA, 2008). In this study, women living in other provinces were more likely to be infected with HIV than those living in the Luanda metropolitan region. However, data on place of birth and residence point in different directions, with place of birth in other provinces appearing as a protective factor while residence in the same provinces appears as a risk factor. This may be due to the small sample size as well as a possible selection bias, with consequent interpretative limitations. On the other hand, taking into account the location, it is legitimate to consider that the general downturn in the economy, the migration of the

rural population to the cities, and the consequent overload on health care, may restrict access to health services in the provinces. This factor, coupled with the technical-resolution limitations in those places, may contribute to the high percentage of women who go to Luanda in search of specialized prenatal medical care. The nature of the data available does not allow us to conclude whether these women are representative of their populations of origin. The same can be said for women from other provinces. Furthermore, several studies have shown an association between place of residence and HIV, emphasizing the internalization of the epidemic (BRITO et al, 2000; VARELLA, 2006;
MUULA, 2008); BRASIL, 2010; NETO et al, 2010; REIS et al., 2008; BRITO2001), a fact that in the present study was evidenced in the Umbundo ethnic group.

As for the association between ethnicity and HIV, most studies define it according to the definition of ethnicity, which does not legitimize a coherent discussion of the current findings. In the present study, ethnicity was defined according to the national language spoken, highlighting the "Bantu" ethnic origin from which around 90% of the Angolan population originates (REDINHA, 1984; LUKOMBO, (1997; FERNANDES, and NTONDO, 2002; SANTOS, 2007). There was a greater chance of infection for the Umbundo ethnic group and for foreigners (Creole and French). No references were found regarding the ethnic distribution of HIV in Angola, which limits this discussion.

Although the high prevalence of HIV in neighboring countries and border regions (Belgian and Democratic Congo, Zimbabwe, Zambia) may put Angola at risk (PNLS, 1997; MINISTÉRIO DA SAÚDE DE ANGOLA, 2009; WHO 2009), women of the Kicongo ethnic group had the same chance of infection as those of the Kimbundo ethnic group. It is believed that this difference in relation to neighboring countries may be related to possible behavioral, cultural and religious differences that offer protective mechanisms such as reduced number of partners and polygamy dissociated from promiscuity, making the Kicong less exposed to HIV infection. This pattern of behavior is probably due to the migratory flow in the border regions of Angola which occurred under the influence of evangelical churches (Baptists, Methodists, Congregationalists and Adventists) in transmitting models of Western culture, (REDINHA, 1984; NETO, 1997; LUKOMBO, 1997; FERNANDES, and NTONDO, 2002; SANTOS, 2007).

Socio-economic factors according to the productive integration of women and heads of household

In the block of socio-economic variables, schooling and personal spending were associated with HIV in the univariate analysis, but did not remain in the final intra-block model.

Occupation represents an individual socio-economic indicator, reflecting aspects such as schooling, income, living conditions, housing and sanitation, among others, which in turn can predispose to unfavorable conditions and consequent vulnerability to HIV infection (CASSANO et al, 2000; KONOPKA, et al, 2010). Although the increased chance of becoming infected with HIV seen in housewives was not statistically significant in relation to the comparison group in this case, it is not exempt from the probable close relationship between HIV and the conditions mentioned above due to female vulnerability centered on heterosexuality (CASSANO et al, 2000); BRITO et al, 2000; SANTOS and OLIVEIRA, 2009; KONOPKA, et al, 2010). In this case, studies into the possible association between HIV and unpaid work in the home are necessary, since many studies point to gender vulnerability for HIV infection by emphasizing that women in male-dominated cultural environments, rarely question their partner's behavior and hardly make demands that could interfere with the male prerogative of enjoying sex free of responsibility (HEILBORN, 1999), especially when associated with unpaid household work (KONOPKA, et al, 2010). and consequent difficulties in accessing resources and opportunities that modify preventive behaviors (SANTOS and OLIVEIRA, 2009; KONOPKA, et al, 2010 ; BRITO et al, 2000; CASSANO et al, 2000). On the other hand, schooling is shown to be protective because it represents a differentiator, which could be education? school environment? Further studies could probably shed more light on the association between schooling and HIV in this population.

As for the income of the women studied, the data do not point to a clear association with infection. Women with some income had an increased chance of infection. The protective effect of women who reported having no income contrasts with the local conditions of poverty and extreme poverty of around 68% and 26% respectively, where individuals survive on less than 2 dollars a day (RIBEIRO, 2007), as an indicator of the impoverishment of the epidemic (; SANTOS, et al 2002; SILVEIRA et al, 2008; SANTOS et al. 2009; NETO, et al, 2010; JUNIOR, 1995; (MUULA, 2008).

Although the income of the head of the household proved to be protective for the women studied when compared to those who declared that the head of the household had no income, this may be considered an epidemiologically plausible finding given the profile of poverty, low schooling and seroprevalence that are significant for the epidemiological scenario of HIV in this sub-Saharan region of Africa (RIBEIRO, 2007; MACHAVA, 2007; MUULA, 2008); MACHAVA, 2007; MUULA, 2008). The protective effect of declared income in relation to heads of household seems to highlight the socio-economic dependence of these women (RIBEIRO, 2007) and their increased vulnerability as an independent socio-economic risk factor for HIV. Studies carried out on the African continent report high rates of poverty and unemployment among women. Seventy percent of the female population in Mogambique is unemployed (MACHAVA, 2007), 68% in Angola (RIBEIRO, 2007) and 40% in South Africa (MUULA, 2008). Finally, the analysis of the group of socio-economic variables according to women's productive insertion and heads of household suggests that women who have a higher income have an increased chance of HIV. On the other hand, when the income of the head of household is higher, the chance of infection is lower. This association suggests that women with higher incomes have greater autonomy and are therefore more likely to be exposed to HIV.

Socio-economic factors according to women's consumption patterns

As for the consumption patterns of the women studied, the statistically significant association between the type of housing, water supply and possession of household goods points to unfavorable socio-economic conditions, which is in line with the findings of PARPINELLI, et al (2000); PAULO (2004); SILVA (2005), precarious local basic sanitation (, PAULO, 2004; SILVA, 2005; UNDP, 2008), as situations associated with increased vulnerability to HIV. Data from the country reveals that of the 53% of the population living with acceptable sanitation conditions, only 62% (urban) and 39% (rural) consumed drinking water (Human Development Report, UNDP, 2008). Houses built with zinc sheets and pau-a-pic (mud, water and wood) represent an increased chance of HIV infection. Although masonry housing has been defined as housing made of cement blocks, bricks, sand and cement, this does not in itself measure good housing or socio-economic conditions, since this material (for construction) is available to the majority of the population, regardless of their purchasing power. The increased chance of HIV among women associated with the possession of household goods and the supply of drinking water through cisterns and standpipes suggests that the better the social conditions, the greater the demand for possession of goods and, consequently, the closer the conditions of vulnerability to HIV. This result recalls the initial epidemiological aspect of HIV among individuals with greater purchasing power, thus revoking the impoverishment that current studies have pointed to (BRASÍL, 2006, LOPES et al, 2007), which observed the restriction of access to goods, strongly associated with the event. Thus, the analysis of the results of this block points in two different directions: on the one hand, the greater the possession of consumer goods, the greater the chance of infection, suggesting that women with a higher standard of living increase their risk of HIV. On the other hand, the data on housing and water suggest that worse living conditions are associated with a greater chance of infection. In view of this finding, it is important to admit the possibility of an association between personal income and the ownership of consumer goods, especially when it is noted that for women with no income or with an income of up to 300 dollars, 10% of them own 6 or more goods, and this percentage increases to 32% when personal income exceeds 300 dollars. These data seem to reinforce the idea that higher income is linked to greater ownership of assets and possibly greater autonomy and greater risk of infection. But what can be concluded is that the relationship between social status and HIV is not direct, highlighting the importance of knowing how cultural and behavioral factors can interact with socioeconomic conditions and directly influence the risk of infection.

Political factors

Some studies emphasize that mobility, migration, social upheaval due to wars and political instability interact with poverty and can condition increased vulnerability to HIV/AIDS (AYRES, 1994; SWEAT and DENISON, 1995; TAWIL et al., 1995; TURSHEN, 1995; AGGLETON, 1996; CARAEL et al., 1997). In the present study, the analysis of variables related to the country's political situation suggests an independent association with HIV infection. However, the small sample size limits the interpretation of the results of this block.

CONCLUSIONS AND SUGGESTIONS

The association between HIV and age suggests an increased prevalence of infection after the age of 30 and consequently underreporting in younger women, implying that women's health policies should be aimed at this group and that voluntary HIV testing should be encouraged before pregnancy.

The Umbundo ethnic group showed the highest association with HIV.

Although this is the largest ethnic representation in the country, more studies are needed to identify behavioral and cultural differences that may show an association with HIV in the various ethnic population representations.

Socio-economic status showed no clear association with HIV infection, suggesting a double pattern, thus highlighting the complexity of the network of infection determinants.

ARTICLE 2* - Association between cultural factors and sexual transmission of HIV in pregnant women

Association between cultural factors and sexual transmission of HIV in pregnant women

ABSTRACT: Introduction: HIV infection in women is on the increase worldwide. Cultural aspects contribute to increasing women's vulnerability to sexual transmission of HIV. Objectives: To identify cultural factors associated with HIV infection in Angolan women. Method: A case-control study was carried out involving 1092 pregnant women, of whom 273 were cases (women with positive HIV serology) and 819 were controls (women with negative HIV serology), selected from prenatal care at the Augusto Ngangula maternity hospital in Luanda, Angola, between 2007 and 2009. Results: Cultural factors were independently associated with HIV infection. Women with two or more previous marital relationships (OR=5.39, IC95%, p= 0.000) who were victims of psychological violence (OR=12.58, IC95%, p=0.000), who lived in polygamous unions (OR=0.30; 7.91; 3.45, IC95%, p=0.043; who took the initiative to start an affective relationship (OR=4.52 , IC95%, p=0.000) had a higher chance of HIV infection. Conclusions: The results show that the sexuality of Angolan women suggests a strong gender hierarchy and that cultural barriers make it difficult for society to be more open to aspects related to sexual and reproductive health being incorporated into actions to prevent and control the expansion of the HIV/AIDS epidemic.

Key Words: HIV, AIDS, sexual transmission, pregnant women, risk factors, cultural factors

Association between cultural and sexual factors and HIV infection in pregnant women

SUMMARY: Background: HIV infection in the female population is expanding worldwide. Cultural aspects may contribute to increased vulnerability of women to sexual transmission of HIV. Objectives: To identify cultural factors associated with HIV infection in Angolan women. Methods: A case control study was conducted, comprising 1092 pregnant women of which 273 were cases (women who were seropositive for HIV) and 819 were controls (women who were seronegative for HIV), selected from the antenatal maternity Ngangula of Luanda-Angola in the period 2007 to 2009. Results: Cultural factors were independently associated with HIV infection. Women with two or more previous marital relationships (OR=5.39 , IC95%, p= 0.000), victims of psychological (OR=12.58 , IC95%, p=0.000), who lived in polygamous unions (OR=0.30; 7.91; 3.45, IC95%, p=0.043; and who took the initiative to the beginning of the affective relationship (OR=4.52 , IC95%, p=0.000) had increased chance of HIV infection. CONCLUSION: The results show that women's sexuality in Angola is marked by strong hierarchy of gender and cultural barriers that hinder greater openness of society to the incorporation of issues related to the sexual and reproductive health into the prevention and control of the spread of HIV / AIDS

Keywords: HIV, sexual transmission, pregnant women, risk factors, cultural factors

INTRODUCTION

In recent times, the incidence of HIV infection among women has increased rapidly and in significant numbers throughout the world (UNAIDS, 2009). Of the 33 million people infected with HIV/AIDS in 2007, approximately 50% were women, making it the fourth leading cause of death among women of working age (UNAIDS 2007). In sub-Saharan Africa, WHO estimates indicate that the situation is even more serious. Of the 5.6 million infected individuals, 3 million, more than half, are women, far exceeding the number of infected women in the rest of the world. Specifically in Angola, the number of adults living with HIV at the end of 2009 was 166,900 individuals, of which 100,931 were women (UNAIDS 2010).

This shift in the path of the epidemic towards feminization around the world has led to a proportionality of the disease between men and women, determined by the increase in the number of infected heterosexuals (UNAIDS Report, 2008). In countries where HIV is spread mainly through heterosexual intercourse, sexual intercourse without the use of condoms is the main risk behavior perceived by women in terms of their personal vulnerability, without, however, being enough to determine changes in behavior.

Similarly, in Angola, sexual transmission between heterosexual couples is responsible for the majority of HIV cases (INLS, 2005; JOÃO 2005; PRATA et al, 2005; MONTEIRO, 2009) due to the non-use of condoms. This refers not only to the demographic, political, socioeconomic and behavioral aspects involved in this issue, but mainly to the concepts of vulnerability, devaluation and subjection of women, culturally defined (LOFORTE, 2007; DEGREGORI et al., 2007) in this country, increasing the individual (MONTEIRO, 2009) or collective risk of contracting HIV infection.

In this context, men and women act in a cultural environment that establishes gender relations, habits, customs and behaviors marked by inequalities (DEGREGORI et al., 2007). This inequality of power unfavorable to women, based on patriarchal foundations, makes them invisible and thus incapable of negotiating rights (SAFFIOTI, 1987), in this case sexual and reproductive rights, increasing their risk of becoming infected and infecting others with HIV (SILVA & VARGENS, 2009; BUCHALLA & PAIVA, 2002; SALDANHA, 2005; WERNECK, 2005).

Cultural peculiarities such as polygamy (male sexual multipartnership), circumcision, widow inheritance and the sexual violation of virgin girls (KALIPENI, et AL., 2007), abominable practices in the context of the rational and especially the feminine, are also among the influential behavioral factors in the growing HIV/AIDS epidemic and contribute to keeping women more submissive and inferior (RUSHING, 1995; SHANNON et al., 1991; OPPONG and KALIPENI, 1999) in Africa.

Studies carried out in African countries show that, due to culturally defined values, communication between couples is an uncommon practice, with men being responsible for making decisions in the context of conjugal relationships on issues relating to reproduction and contraception (DEGREGORI et al., 2007). This dynamic in relationships between men and women makes it difficult to adopt prevention measures based on condom use, which would require negotiation between partners.

METHODOLOGY

This is a case-control study involving 1092 pregnant women, 273 cases and 819 controls, selected during prenatal consultations at the Augusto Ngangula maternity hospital in Luanda, Angola, between 2007 and 2009. This institution is a national reference for the Ministry of Health and the Agostinho Neto University for medical care, including the vertical transmission of HIV/AIDS in pregnant women and teaching activities at postgraduate level. Women who tested positive or negative for HIV, respectively, when submitted to the rapid test, were considered cases or controls. All ethical requirements were met, as well as submission to and approval by the ethics committees for research involving human beings at the Federal University of Pernambuco, in Brazil, and the Angolan Ministry of Health.

The data collection technique was an individual interview, carried out in a private consultation room, using a questionnaire made up of closed questions, applied by the main researcher. A pilot study was carried out to help estimate the sample size and adapt the data collection instrument. The database was built using the EPI-INFO 6.0 statistical program and the data was analyzed using the STATA 9.0 statistical package. Initially, a univariate analysis was carried out, checking the association of each variable with HIV infection. The Odds Ratio (OR) was calculated with the respective 95% confidence intervals and the corresponding "p" value. Variables with a p-value of <0.20 in the association with the outcome were entered into a multivariate model. In the multivariate stage of the analysis, the variables with a p-value of <0.05 remained in the final model.

The variables studied were: partner's age, partner's controlling behavior, physical, psychological and/or sexual violence inflicted by the partner, physical violence by other family members, history of marital separation in the current relationship, previous marital union experience, living in a polygamous relationship, initiative to start the relationship and having a religion.

The approach to violence was based on the questions used in the World Health Organization's Multi-Country Study on Health and Domestic Violence (GARCIA-MORENO et al , 2005), validated in Portuguese (Brazil) by Schraiber et al (SCHRAIBER ET Al, 2010). These made it possible to identify physical, sexual and psychological violence and controlling behaviors perpetrated by the intimate partners of the women studied. Thus, physical violence was characterized by acts of physical aggression or the use of objects or weapons to produce injuries; psychological violence, by threatening behaviour, humiliation or insults; sexual violence, by the reporting of sexual relations by means of physical force or threats and the imposition of acts considered humiliating by the women. A detailed description of the issues has already been published by other authors (SCHRAIBER ET AL, 2007; LUDERMIR ET AL, 2010). An operational definition was created for the variable physical violence inflicted by other family members, using the WHO definition as a reference (GARCIA-MORENO et al., 2005). Violence was considered when the woman answered yes to at least one of the questions.

RESULTS

Of the total of 1092 women involved in the study, 273 represented the cases and 819 the controls. With regard to the characteristics of the relationship with the partner, it was found that 79.67% of the women had been initiated into an affective relationship by their partner, 93.04% had never left home as a form of temporary separation and 25.55% had had more than two marital experiences. The partners were predominantly aged between 30 and 39 and 34.8% reported having a polygamous relationship (table 1).

In the univariate analysis, the variables initiative for an affective relationship, temporary separation, previous marital union, partner's age and living in a polygamous relationship showed a statistically significant association with HIV infection (Table 1).

Table 1 - Distribution of cases and controls according to the number of previous marriages and initiative to start a relationship.

Variables	Case	%	Control	%	Total	%	OR	(95% CI)	p
Union previous One	107	39.19	706	86.20	813	74.45	1	-	-
Two/more	166	60.81	113	13.80	279	25.55		9.69 (7.08-13.27)	0.000
Initiative from relado Man	140	51.28	730	89.13	870	79.67	1	-	-
Woman	133	48.72	89	10.87	222	20.33	7.79	5.64- 10.77	0.000

Table 2- Distribution of cases and controls according to religion and age of partner.

Variables	Case	%	Control	%	Total	%		OR	(95% CI)	p

Religion									
With religion.	263	96.34	778	94.99	1,041	95.33	1	-	-
No religion.	10	3.66	41	5.01	51	4.67	0.72	(0.36- 1.46)	0.364
Agepartner									
o(years)									
20 a 29	51	18.68	327	39.93	378	34.62	1	-	-
30 a 39	153	56.04	377	46.03	530	48.53	2.60	(1.83-3.69)	0.000
40 and over	62	22.71	97	11.84	159	14.56	4.10	(2.65-6.33)	0.000
You don't know	7	2.56	18	2.20	25	2.29	2.49	(0.99- 6.27)	0.052

Table 3- Distribution of cases and controls according to polygamy and <u>temporary</u> marital separation <u>in the current report.</u>

Variables	Case	%	Control	%	Total	%	OR	(95% CI)	P
Polygamy It doesn't	123	45.05	587	71.67	710	65.02	1	-	-
another There's another	9	3.30	146	17.83	155	14.19	0.29	(0.15- 0.59)	0.001

It has 2 to 4	112	41.03	48	5.86	160	14.65	11.14	(7.54-16.45)	0.000
women > 5	29	10.62	38	4.64	67	6.14	3.64	(2.16- 6.13)	0.000
Temporary separation Never	235	86.08	781	95.36	1,016	93.04	1	-	-
Yes	38	13.92	38	4.64	76	6.96	3.32 (2.07-5.33)		0.000

The controlling behavior of the partner was mentioned by 7.69% of the women and 7.42% reported having suffered psychological violence (table 2).

Table 4 - Distribution of cases and controls according to controlling behavior by the partner (CCP), psychological, physical and sexual violence by the partner and physical violence by other family members

Violence	Case	Control	Total	OR	IC	P
CCP						
No	213(78,02)	795(97,07)	1,008(92,31)	1		
Yes	60(21,98)	24(2,93)	84(7,69)	9,33	5,68-15,34	0,000
Psycholog.						
No	212(77,66)	799(97,56)	1,011(92,58)	1		

Yes	61(22,34)	20(2,44)	81(7,42)	11,50	6,78-9,48	0,000
Physics						
No	235(86,08)	791(96,58)	1,026(93,96)	1	-	-
Yes	38(13,92)	28(3,42)	66(6,04)	4,57	2,74-7,60	0,000
Sexual						
No	265(97,07)	818(99,88)	1,083(99,18)	1		
Yes	8(2,93)	1(0,12)	9(0,82)	24,69	3,07-198,32	0,003

In the multivariate analysis, all the variables related to the partner's controlling behavior and violence also showed a statistically significant association with the outcome. After reciprocal adjustment, only the variables initiative for the affective relationship, number of marital unions, having suffered psychological violence inflicted by the partner and living in polygamous relationships remained in the final intra-block model (table 3).

Table 5- Association between HIV and cultural risk factors in women - M ANG , 2007 a 2008, Luanda-Angola

Variable	Study population		Odds Ratio *			Odds Ratio **		
Initiative of	Case	Control	OR	IC	P	OR	IC	P

relations hip Man Woman	140 (51,28) 133	730 (89,13) 89 (10,87)	1 7,79	5,63-10,77	0,000	4,52	3,00- 6,81	0,000
Union previous marital One Two/mor e	(48,72) 107 (39,19) 166	706 (86,20) 113 (13,80)	1 9,69	6,08-13,27	0,000	5,39	3,67-7,92	0,000
Polygam y No 1 woman	(60,81) 123 (45,05) 9 (3,30)	587 (71,67) 146 (17,83)	1 0,29	0,15-0,59	0,001	0,30	0,14- 0,66	0,043
2 to 4 women	112	48 (5,86)	11,13	7,54-16,45	0,000	7,91	4,96-12,61	0,000
>5 women	(41,03) 29 (10,62)	38 (4,64)	3,64	2,16- 6,13	0,000	3,45	1,87- 6,36	0,000
Psycholo gical violence No Yes	212 (77,66) 61 (22,34)	799 (97,56) 20 (2,44)	1 11,46	6,78- 19,48	0,000	12,58	6,67-23,75	0,000

*** Odds Ratio: univariate analysis; ** Odds Ratio: multivariate analysis; Women's sexual behavior:**

partner's serological status, number of partners, why they don't use condoms, occasional partner, sex under the influence of drugs.

DISCUSSION

Women with two or more previous marital relationships, victims of psychological violence, living in polygamous relationships and those who took the initiative to start an affective relationship had a higher chance of HIV infection. Other studies have shown that cultural diversity can introduce specificities in the way risk factors for HIV infection are expressed in different populations (COHEN and TRUSSELL, 1996; FONSECA and LUCAS, 2009; DIAS S. et al, 2001; BRADBY and WILLIAMS, 1999).

The fact that the woman took the initiative to start the relationship increased the chance of HIV infection, when compared to women in marriages in which other family members were involved. Although this finding suggests greater freedom for women, their marital fidelity may be questionable in the light of the culture still in force in most Angolan families. According to Junior (1995), in Angola, there have always been different ways of starting and formalizing a relationship or marital union within a standardized socio-cultural conduct (from the declaration to start a relationship, to the union by cohabitation or marriage).

On the other hand, the initiative for greater sexual freedom runs counter to the cultural norms of relationships marked by gender hierarchies that still prevail on the African continent. According to a review by Monteiro (2009), although in urban areas of some African countries, young, middle-class women with a higher level of education have been challenging social and moral norms and values in order to experience sexuality more freely, the value "of ideals of purity (virginity)" and control of women's sexuality persists in Africa at the time of marriage. Women who don't meet these requirements tend to make any affective relationship easier (JUNIOR, 1995; MONTEIRO, 2009).

Women who have had more than one marital experience throughout their lives are more likely to be infected with HIV. Several studies have already associated the increased chance of HIV infection with multiple sexual partnerships without the use of safe prevention methods (COHEN and TRUSSELL, 1996; FONSECA and LUCAS, 2009; DIAS S. et al, 2001; BRADBY and WILLIAMS, 1999).

Polygamy, officially practiced in most African countries as a symbol of male power (MAKINWA-ADEBUSOYE, 2002), including in Angola, has been shown to be independently associated with HIV infection. This study draws attention to the fact that this peculiar variant of marital arrangement and expression of sexuality in Angola can expose women to a very high risk of HIV infection in stable marital relationships (PEN DST/HIV/SIDA, 1999; ANGOLA, 2001; PRATA, et, al, 2005). In contrast to multi-partnership, in which extramarital sexual relations involving other women predominate, traditional African polygamy represents the act of maintaining a conjugal relationship with more than one partner, conferring on all the status of wife, with the man assuming the role of provider and the commitment to fidelity, among other obligations. This contradicts some studies in African countries which have shown an inversely significant relationship between HIV/AIDS rates and polygamy rates (KALIPENI, et al, 2007). However, other studies carried out on the

African continent point to polygamy as a risk factor for HIV infection (PEN DST/HIV/SIDA, 1999; ANGOLA, 2001; MAKINWA-ADEBUSOYE, 2002). In the population studied, polygamous unions are associated with a greater chance of HIV infection in unions with three or more women. At the same time, and contradictorily, the findings of this study show a lower chance of HIV infection for women in polygamous marriages with fewer (two) or more (five or more) women. There is evidence that some African men married in monogamous or polygamous relationships have extramarital affairs as a way of asserting their power and masculinity (MAKINWA-ADEBUSOYE, 2002). A study in an African country showed that 20% of HIV-infected women live in stable relationships and have multiple sexual partners as their main source of infection (ALLEN et al, 1991). The scarcity of research investigating the dynamics of relationships in polygamous unions in Angola limits a more accurate interpretation of this finding and suggests the need for additional studies on the power relations between men and women and the experience of sexuality in the context of polygamy.

In Angola, cultural and traditional factors may also contribute to violence being part of Angolan women's way of life. In the population studied, the most frequent form of intimate partner violence was psychological violence, followed by physical violence or violence by other family members, and there was an increased chance of HIV infection in women who reported these types of violence. It is possible that the estimates of the occurrence of violence in its different forms in this study are underestimated due to the embarrassment and fear of reporting violence on the part of some women, as it is a "sensitive" subject that involves aspects of private life that are difficult to declare, especially in quantitative surveys (SCHRAIBER, et, al, 2009).

According to BREITH (1993), gender violence forms a single body with structural injustices and feeds the prevailing logic of a violent culture where the domination of some over others is installed as a natural way of life and ideological support for a society of subordination. HEISE (1994) concludes that violence is "an extremely complex phenomenon, with deep roots in power relations based on gender, sexuality, self-identity and social institutions" and that "in many societies, the (male) right to dominate women is considered the essence of masculinity. This aspect reinforces the idea that addressing partner violence necessarily requires confronting gender inequalities, where sexual relationships stand out as a field of struggle structured fundamentally by the recurring power differences between men and women. Studies show that many women endure abusive relationships and remain in a position of worthlessness, isolation and submission to the abuse they suffer for reasons ranging from maintaining a permanent family union, financial dependence on their partners to a lack of family and community support and, above all, because they are unaware of their rights (CARDOSO, 1997A, 1997B; LAIRD, 2002; MASON, 2002; NARVAZ, and KOLLER, 2006). Studies that have focused on violence in affective-sexual relationships associate greater exposure to HIV with women's lack of control over their sexual and reproductive lives, male supremacy and violence, which is considered to be a right of men (DUNKLE, et al., 2004; BANCHS, 1996, BREITH, 1993; RODRÍGUEZ, 1998). In South Africa, pregnant women with a positive history of partner violence and subjection to predominantly male-controlled sexual relationships were at greater risk of HIV infection (DUNKLE et al., 2004). Similarly, JEWKES et al, (2010), in a cohort study, found that intimate partner violence and unequal power between men and women in the relationship increased the risk of HIV infection in South African women.

CONCLUSIONS AND SUGGESTIONS

The conclusion is that reducing female vulnerability to the HIV/AIDS epidemic presupposes the establishment of public policies and inter-sectoral actions that take into account the particularities of local cultural systems, socio-economic conditions and access to education and health services.

ARTICLE 3* - Association between behavioral factors and sexual transmission of HIV in pregnant women

SUMMARY

Introduction: Sexual intercourse is the main route of HIV transmission. Behavioral factors can increase individual risk for sexual transmission of this virus, especially when associated with inconsistent condom use. **Objectives: To** identify behavioral factors associated with HIV infection in Angolan women. **Method:** A case-control study was carried out involving 1092 pregnant women, of whom 273 were cases (women with positive HIV serology) and 819 were controls (women with negative HIV serology), selected from prenatal care at the Augusto Ngangula maternity hospital in Luanda, Angola, between 2007 and 2009. **Results:** The following factors showed an independent association with HIV infection: partner serology, number of partners, not using condoms and occasional sexual intercourse and under the influence of alcohol. The following partner characteristics showed an independent association with infection in women: age, schooling, barbershop attendance, alcohol use and length of relationship. **Conclusions:** The findings suggest that there is little room for women to negotiate safe sex, making it necessary, alongside educational interventions, to empower them in order to reduce the asymmetry of relationships. Sexual partners do not seem to adhere to condom use due to prevailing cultural patterns, and it is therefore recommended that we reflect on the cultural patterns that can encourage the spread of HIV through sexual intercourse.

Key Words : HIV, sexual transmission, pregnant women, risk factors, sexual behavior

Association between behavioral factors and HIV infection in pregnant women.

SUMMARY

Background: Sexual intercourse is the main route of HIV transmission in heterosexual relationships. Behavioral factors may increase the risk of HIV infection, especially when associated with inconsistent condom use **Objectives:** To identify behavioral factors associated with HIV infection in Angolan women. **Methods:** A case control study was conducted, comprising 1092 pregnant women of which 273 were cases (women who were seropositive for HIV) and 819 were controls (women who were seronegative for HIV), selected from the antenatal maternity Ngangula of Luanda-Angola in the period 2007 to 2009. **Results:** The following factors showed an independent association with HIV infection: serology partner, number of partners, not using condoms and sex under alcohol's influence. The following characteristics of the partners showed an independent association with infection in women: age, education, attending barbershop, alcohol use and length of time of relationship. **CONCLUSIONS:** The findings suggest that there is little room for women to negotiate safe sex and, thus, that it is necessary, in parallel to educational interventions, the empowerment of those women aiming to reduce the asymmetry of the relationship with their partners. Sexual partners do not seem to adhere to condom use due to the current cultural patterns; it is recommended, therefore, to rethink the cultural patterns that may facilitate the spread of HIV through sexual intercourse.

Keywords: HIV, sexual transmission, pregnant women, risk factors, sexual behavioral

INTRODUCTION

Sexual intercourse is the main route of HIV transmission (ALLEN et al. 1991; COHEN, 2002) worldwide (UNAIDS, 2007). Although the risk of transmission from an isolated act of sexual intercourse with an infected person is not precisely known, some studies report the possibility of people who have had several sexual contacts with an infected person without acquiring the virus, while others have become infected following a single sexual encounter. In general, the likelihood of a person acquiring an STD is proportional to the number of sexual partners they have had in previous years. Many studies have shown a significant association between HIV and risk behaviors, such as professional and/or unprotected sex and injecting drug use, among other factors (SINGER, 1994; SOSKOLNE, 2002); (O'DONNELL et al., 2001); (PETTIFOR et al., 2004); (BEADNELL et al., 2005), highlighting the increased vulnerability of women to infection (SILVEIRA et al., 2002). On the other hand, since HIV is not a disease exclusive to prostitutes and sexually promiscuous individuals, other factors, such as gender inequality, can make it difficult for women to protect themselves from infection. African studies show an HIV prevalence of around 20% among low-risk women, considering the only source of exposure to HIV to be the stable male partner who has sexual contacts outside the main relationship (ALLEN et al., 1991).

Gender inequality, cultural, political and socioeconomic peculiarities can shape behavior and increase vulnerability to infection (SILVA and VARGENS, 2009; BUCHALLA and PAIVA, 2002; SALDANHA, 2005; WERNECK, 2005; SILVEIRA et al., 2002). Given the worldwide growth of HIV in the female population and the magnitude of the problem on the African continent, it is essential to identify the behavioral factors that can increase the individual risk of infection in Angolan women, which is the aim of this study.

METHODOLOGY

This article is part of a case-control study to investigate risk factors for the sexual transmission of HIV. A total of 1082 pregnant women were selected for prenatal care at a reference maternity hospital in the city of Luanda, capital of Angola. 273 pregnant women with HIV (cases) were compared to 819 without HIV (controls). All ethical requirements were met, as well as submission to and approval by the ethics committees for research involving human beings at UFPE - Brazil and MINSA - Angola. Data was collected through individual interviews, in a private environment, using a structured form, applied by the researcher after a pilot study to help estimate the sample size and adapt the collection instrument. The data collected allowed for the construction of a database in the EPI-INFO statistical program and analysis using the STATA 8.2 statistical package (Copyright 1984-2003). For analysis, the variables were grouped into blocks. Initially, a univariate analysis was carried out, checking the association of each variable with HIV infection. The odds ratios and respective 95% confidence intervals and p-values were calculated. Variables with a p-value < 0.20 in the association with the outcome were included in an intra-block multivariate model, and those with a p-value < 0.05 remained in this model. This article analyzes and discusses the behavioral risk factors associated with HIV in the women studied, as well as the characteristics and behavior of their partners.

<u>RESULTS</u>

Of the total of 1092 pregnant women involved in the study, 273 represented the cases and 819 the controls. The sample consisted mainly of Angolan women (98.2%), married (94.7%) and aged between 15 and 49. The vast majority (74.8%) had their first sexual intercourse between the ages of 15 and 19 and 99.5% did not use condoms. It was identified that 63.00% of these women had never used any contraceptive method. In the previous 5 years, 98.2% of these women had only had sex with a steady partner and 36.6% had only had one sexual partner. A small number (0.9%) had sex in exchange for favors or reported being sex workers (0.6%). As for the seropositivity of the partner, 8.6% of the cases had HIV-positive partners while 58.8% were unaware of their partner's serological status.

In the behavioral factors block, all the variables relating to women showed a statistically significant association with HIV infection in the univariate analysis. In the multivariate analysis, the following variables remained in the model: the serological status of the partner, the number of sexual partners, non-use of condoms, sexual intercourse with an occasional partner and sexual intercourse under the influence of alcohol (table 1).

Table 1- Association between women's sexual behavior (serology and number of partners) and HIV infection in women - M ANG , 2007 to 2008, Luanda-Angola

Variable	Study population		Odds Ratio *			Odds Ratio **		
Serology	**Case**	**Control**	**OR**	**IC**	**P**	**OR**	**IC**	**P**
HIV-	52(19.05)	309(37.73)	1	-	-	-	-	-

Variable	Case	Control	OR	IC	P	OR	IC	P
HIV+	81(29.67)	7(0.85)	68.76	30.10-157.08	0.000	48.60	18.27-29.34	0.000
don't know	140(51.28)	503(61.42)	1.65	1.17-2.34	0.005	1.59	0.96-2.64	0.074
Partners								
1 parcel	27(9.89)	373(45.54)	1		-	-	-	-
2 parcels	40(14.65)	276(33.70)	2.00	1.20-3.34	0.008	1.70	0.87-3.33	0.122
3 parcels	94(34.43)	124(15.14)	10.47	6.52-16.82	0.000	6.37	3.40-11.93	0.000
4 parc e +	112(41.03)	46(5.62)	33.65	19.99-56.56	0.000	12.42	6.01-25.67	0.000

*** Odds Ratio: univariate analysis; ** Odds Ratio: multivariate analysis; Women's sexual behavior: partner's serological status, number of partners, why they don't use condoms, occasional partner, sex under the influence of drugs.**

Table - 2: Association between women's sexual behavior and HIV infection in women - M ANG , 2007 to 2008, Luanda-Angola.

Variable	Study population		Odds Ratio *			Odds Ratio **		
PNUPPF	Case	Control	OR	IC	P	OR	IC	P
married	29(10.62)	299(36.51)	1	-	-	-	-	-
use another method	18(6.59)	14(1.71)	13.27	5.98 29.38	0.000	6.34	1.38 29.18	0.018

Variable	Study population		Odds Ratio *			Odds Ratio **		
carelessness	170(62.27)	308(37.61)	5.69	3.72 8.70	0.000	12.00	5.07 28.40	0.000
elenao likes **UPPO***	56(20.51)	198(24.18)	2.92	1.60 4.73	0.000	11.73	4.67 29.46	0.000
No parcoca	99 (36.26)	780(95.24)	1	-	-	-	-	-
Not used	124(45.42)	10(1.22)	97.69697	49.62 192.34	0.000	149.25	56.55 393.93	0.000
used **<u>Sex under alcohol</u>**	50(18.32)	29(3.54)	13.58	8.21 22.46	0.000	18.07	7.36 44.38	0.000
No	235(86.08)	769(93.89)	1	-	-	-	-	-
Yes	38(13.92)	50(6.11)	2.49	1.59 3.87	0.000	0.08	0.03-0.22	0.000

*** Odds Ratio: univariate analysis; ** Odds Ratio: multivariate analysis; Women's sexual behavior: partner's serological status, number of partners, why they don't use condoms, occasional partner, sex under the influence of drugs. UPPO*** condom use with occupational partner. PNUPPF: why not using a condom with a steady partner**

As for the characteristics and behaviors of the partners, age, frequent visits to the barber, alcohol use, schooling and length of time living with the partner showed an independent association with HIV infection (Table 2).

Table 3: Association between partner characteristics (age, barbering, alcohol consumption) and HIV infection in women - M ANG , 2007 to 2008 , Luanda-Angola

Variable	Study population	Odds Ratio *	Odds Ratio **

Age#	Case	Control	OR	IC	P	OR	IC	P
20-29	51(18.68)	327(39.93)	1	-	-	-	-	-
30-49	153(56.04)	374(46.03)	2.60	1.83-3.69	0.000	3.11	2.11- 4.58	0.000
49 >	62(22.71)	97(11.84)	4.10	2.65-6.33	0.000	5.73	3.47-9.45	0.000
You don't know	7(2.56)	18(2.20)	2.49	0.99-6.27	0.052	4.50	1.67-12.11	0.003
Barber no	95 (34.80)	469 (57.26)	1	-	-	-	-	-
yes	178 (65.20)	350(42.74)	2.51	1.89-3.34	0.000	2.31	1.70-3.15	0.000
Alcohol no	173 (63.37)	374 (45.67)	1	-	-	-	-	-
yes	160(58.6)	412(50.3)	2.06	1.55-2.73	0.000	1.72	1.26-2.35	0.001

* Odds Ratio ; ** Odds Ratio # age in years

Table 2.2: Association between partner characteristics (schooling and length of time living with partner) and HIV infection in women - M ANG , 2007 to 2008 , Luanda-Angola

Variable	Study population		Odds Ratio *			Odds Ratio **		
School rity	Case	Control	OR	IC	P	OR	IC	P
Fund	32 (11.72)	35 (4.27)	1	-	-	-	-	-
Medium	99 (36.26)	313 (38.22)	0.35	0.20-0.59	0.000	0.45	0.24- 0.77	0.004
Superior	34 (12.45)	79 (9.65)	0.47	0.25- 0.88	0.018	0.47	0.23- 0.93	0.031
You don't know	108(39.56)	392(47.86)	0.30	0.18-0.51	0.000	0.29	0.16- 0.52	0.000
Tconv#								
<1 year	32(11.72)	122(14.90)	1	-	-	-	-	-
1 a 5	161(58.97)	300(36.63)	2.05	1.33-3.16	0.000	1.75	1.09-2.82	0.021
>5 years	69(25.27)	318(38.83)	0.83	0.52-1.32	0.427	0.48	0.27- 0.82	0.006
You don't know	11(4.03)	79(9.65)	0.53	0.25-1.11	0.094	0.43	0.20-0.94	0.036

*** Odds Ratio ; ** Odds Ratio # time living with partner**

DISCUSSION
Women's sexual behavior

The study of risk behavior for HIV infection in Angolan women pointed to the importance of the serological status of the partner, the number of sexual partners, the use of condoms with a steady or occasional partner and the practice of sexual intercourse under the influence of alcohol. As for the characteristics and behavior of the partners, the age and schooling of the partner, the frequency of barbering, the use of alcohol and the length of time living with the partner showed an independent association with HIV infection. The behavioral factors indicating risk in this study are in line with other studies (SILVEIRA, et al., 2002). (MINISTÉRIO DA SAÚDE, 2002); (SEIDMAN et al., 1994; ALAN, 1998; OLINTO e GALVÄO,1999; SHEPHERD et al., 2000), but also point to local specificities.

The serological status of the partners of the women studied showed a statistically significant association with HIV infection, with a higher risk of infection in the group with an HIV-positive partner, as expected. In addition, the finding regarding knowledge of the serology of the partners was noteworthy, as it disagreed with other studies which identified considerably higher proportions of women who knew their partners' serology (SANTOS et al., 2009; GALVÄO et al., 2004).

The strong association with the partner's positivity can be interpreted in two ways:

One possibility could be that the women knew their partner's HIV status before becoming infected and did not take the necessary precautions, since they were pregnant at the time of the interview. According to the literature, some reasons that could lead to this behavior are related to marital submissiveness in the gender relationship, which can make it difficult to negotiate safe sex (SAFFIOTI HIB, 1992; QUINN SC., 1993), as well as to end the marital relationship. Another possibility is that the women became aware of this condition when they were already exposed to HIV and/or pregnant.

Any of the above alternatives suggests inequality of power in affective, marital and/or intimate relationships, leading to difficulties in protecting against HIV (VILLELA, 2008). Many women have little influence over decisions regarding how, when and under what conditions to have sex, a condition which has contributed to the feminization of HIV (JIMENEZ et al., 2001). This situation puts women at risk and has important implications in terms of infection control strategies.

The number of sexual partners showed an independent association with infection. It was found that the risk of becoming infected with HIV increases with the number of partners, thus agreeing with data in the literature (ALLEN et al., 1991; SEIDMAN et al., 1992; SEIDMAN et al., 1994; SILVEIRA et al., 2002). This may be a reflection of a lifetime of choices dependent on submission in a society with significant gender differences.

Having sex without using condoms was an independent risk factor for HIV infection, thus corroborating the fact that consistent condom use is the only efficient method of protection against STD/AIDS in heterosexual relationships, especially when penetration is the most practiced method (DAVIS et al., 1999). Several studies show an incompatibility between preventive rationality and socio-affective rationality when aspects such as length of relationship, type of partner, trust and monogamy, as well as the image of being a good mother/wife, are superimposed, which can contribute to a false sense of security (CHIN, 1999; PRAÇA and GUALDA, 2003; HEBLING and GUIMARÂES, 2004); AMORIM and ANDRADE, 2006; SANTOS and IRIART, 2007). Many women stop worrying about HIV/AIDS, relying on a moral code in which marriage seems to guarantee immunity from the disease, leading to the misinterpretation that only women in extramarital relationships could become infected, and that women with a single partner and a stable relationship, sustained by affection and love, would be protected from infection (ALVES RN et al., 2002; THIENGO, 2005; NASCIMENTO, 2005; GIACOMOZZI and CAMARGO, 2004; GIACOMOZZI and CAMARGO, 2006; SILVA and VARGENS, 2009).

The increased chance associated with careless condom use in stable or occasional relationships is in line with other studies. The authors state that women find it difficult to identify their own risk and that self-perception is not a good indicator of real risk (ALVES et al., 2002; HEBLING and GUIMARAES, 2004); NASCIMENTO and BARBOSA, 2005; THIENGO, 2005; GIACOMOZZI and CAMARGO, 2006; SILVA and VARGENS, 2009); SANTOS and IRIART, 2007; AMORIM and ANDRADE, 2006).

There was a higher risk for women who reported not using condoms because their partner claimed not to like them. This situation has been mentioned by other scholars when they report that many women, although they are aware of the risks of becoming infected with HIV, are forced to give up condoms in order to submit to their partners' wishes, probably as a result of the gender inequality already mentioned throughout this text (SAFFIOTI, 1992; GOGNA, 1997; SILVA, e VARGENS, 2009; BUCHALLA e PAIVA, 2002; SALDANHA, 2005; WERNECK, 2005; SANTOS e IRIART, 2007). In view of this, it can be observed that marital agreements can become more important than self-care and that prevention can be seen as a threat to married life. SIMOES-BARBOSA (1999) identified that, for many women, the loss of social identity as a result of breaking affective, sexual and material ties is more important than the individual risk of HIV infection. This behavior highlights the difficulty in implementing educational measures to control the epidemic.

Inconsistent condom use in sexual relations with an occasional partner proved to be an important risk behavior in the population studied. The lack of adherence pointed out by various authors may be associated with sexual dissatisfaction, loss of trust and intimacy, including discontinuation of the relationship with the partner, outcomes often mentioned by the women surveyed (WORTH, 1989; PIVNICK, 1993), regardless of whether the relationship is fixed or occasional. In addition, women's initiative to practice safe sex can be detrimental to any benefit when the exchange of favors or sex as a source of income is the crucial objective.

Alcohol consumption has been associated with risky sexual behavior for STDs/HIV/AIDS (UNAIDS, 2006; BENOTSCH et al., 2006; CARDOSO et al., 2008). Many studies have reported that the risk behaviors frequently associated with alcohol use before or during sex are the following: casual sex, multiple partners and sex without a condom (SINGER, 1994; MALOW et al., 2001; BACHANAS et al., 2002; DICLEMENTE et al., 2002; GRIFFIN ET AL., 2006; LIU et al., 2006; (CARDOSO et al., 2008); ROBERTS, 2006 ; MSUYA et al., 2006). The association between alcohol consumption and HIV suggested by these studies was initially evidenced in the present study. However, in the multivariate analysis, this variable proved to be protective, suggesting a confounding effect of other variables. This change seems to indicate that the behavioral factors linked to alcohol and the higher risk of infection are represented in the other variables of the model; the change in direction occurred when the variable "use of condoms with occasional partners" was adjusted for, suggesting that the non-use of condoms would be the mechanism mediating this risk. Additional information quantifying alcohol consumption could help to understand this association. Furthermore, the possibility of a spurious association (alpha error) cannot be ruled out. However, the association with alcohol use by partners remains statistically significant.

Partner characteristics and risk behavior

The characteristics and behavior of the partners are related to the risk of them becoming infected and subsequently transmitting the infection to their partners.

The present study found a statistically significant association between the age of the women's partners and HIV infection, as is the case in several African regions. The marital union of women with older partners is in turn associated with socio-economic destabilization, gender inequality, polygamy and domestic violence, among other factors (ANDERSSON et al., 2007; MUULA and ADMSON, 2008; ONUSIDA AND WHO, 2009; KHOBOTLO et al., 2009). The increased risk of HIV infection in women who do not know their partner's age points less to a lack of interest in getting to know them than to cultural factors such as those mentioned above which may be at the root of this type of behavior, thus showing its agreement with other studies (MUULA, 2008 ANGOLA, 2000; MAKINWA-ADEBUSOYE, 2002). In addition to sexual intercourse, the blood-borne route, through transfusion and the use of injectable drugs, represents another important route of HIV contamination in adults. However, transmission by handling sharp instruments, such as those used in barbershops, circumcision centers, facial scarification, tattoos, ear piercing, administration of parenteral medication via IM or IV, beauty salons, among others, has been little reported. In the present study, having a sexual partner with a previous history of cutting hair, shaving and nails in barbershops was considered a risk situation. In this category, as in other studies (GIR, and GESSOLO, 1998; ARULOGUN and ADESORO, 2009), there was a greater chance of HIV infection for the respective women.

The use of alcoholic beverages by the partner showed an association with HIV infection in women, in agreement with previous studies carried out in the United States and Brazil which pointed to an association between the consumption of psychoactive substances and the non-consistent use of condoms (BASTOS et al., 2008; BERTONI et al., 2009).

As for the partner's schooling, the protective effect of higher schooling corroborates some studies which show that a higher level of education is consistent with safer behavior, such as condom use (WALQUE, 2006). Not knowing one's partner's schooling seems to be a proxy for another situation, suggesting an asymmetrical relationship where not even the basic characteristics of partners are known.

As for the length of time living with a steady partner, there are few references available. In this study, living with partners for between 1 and 5 years showed a direct association with HIV infection, while living with them for more than five years or not knowing the time showed an inverse association. A period of more than five years may suggest a steady partner and a stable relationship, although women with shorter periods of cohabitation cannot be excluded from these situations.

CONCLUSIONS AND SUGGESTIONS

The complexity of the issues involved in the dynamics of HIV risk behavior in both women and their partners is evident from the above. Cultural factors led to the conclusion that Angolan women's sexuality is marked by a strong gender hierarchy. Cultural barriers can make it difficult for society to be more open to aspects related to sexual and reproductive health. The behavioral factors found suggest the existence of asymmetrical relationships, lack of adherence to condom use by partners and little space for women to negotiate safe sex.

In view of the above conclusions, it is necessary, in parallel with educational interventions, to empower women to practice safe sex regardless of the stability of their relationships and to minimize asymmetry in marital life; as well as to reflect deeply on the cultural patterns of Angolan society that can encourage the spread of HIV through sexual intercourse.

CONCLUSIONS AND FINAL CONSIDERATIONS

In order to answer the guiding question of this thesis, which risk factors are associated with the sexual transmission of HIV, a literature review and an empirical study were carried out.

The bibliographical research used to support this study revealed that HIV infection among women remains high, especially in the sub-Saharan region of Africa, where underdevelopment and culture have a particular influence on the global statistics of the HIV/AIDS epidemic. This study has allowed us to draw conclusions and prompt further reflection:

- The identification of risk factors for the sexual transmission of HIV in women allowed them to be grouped into different levels of determination: demographic and socioeconomic, cultural and behavioral.

- From a demographic point of view, the association between HIV and age allows us to consider the possibility of an increased prevalence of infection from the age of 30 onwards and, consequently, underreporting in younger women, implying that women's health policies should target this group and encourage voluntary HIV testing before pregnancy. This finding implies increasingly early women's health policies aimed at sexual education and encouraging voluntary HIV testing before pregnancy. Although the Umbundo ethnic group's association with HIV may be due to the fact that it is the largest ethnic group in the country, more studies are needed to identify behavioral and cultural differences that may show an association with HIV in the country's different ethnic groups.

- The socio-economic factors identified do not point to an association in a single direction, but show the complexity of the determinants of the disease.
It also suggests the existence of a double pattern of transmission.

- The results showed that women's sexuality is marked by a strong gender hierarchy associated with cultural barriers that often make it difficult for society to open up to issues related to sexual and reproductive health, which can increase the risk of HIV transmission.

- Polygamy has been shown to be associated with HIV infection. It is noteworthy that this peculiar variant of marital arrangement and expression of sexuality in Angola can expose women to a very high risk of HIV infection in stable marital relationships. On the other hand, women who have had more than one partner throughout their lives and those who take the initiative in a romantic relationship also have an increased chance of infection.

- Further studies are needed to better understand female vulnerability associated with the HIV epidemic, taking into account local cultural models in order to provide appropriate forms of intervention. Maintaining relationships with partners who disagree with condom use, putting women at risk of HIV transmission, suggests gender inequality in relationships, associated with subordinacy and lack of decisive power over sexual life. In this context, it is important not only to promote access to education, information and sexual and reproductive health services, but also to promote educational interventions that lead to the empowerment of women, in order to enable the practice of safe sex regardless of the stability of relationships and to minimize the asymmetry of relationships.

- In order to minimize cultural "taboos" that can make it difficult to change attitudes and behaviors, the participation of health workers from the community itself, who are qualified to communicate and advise on women's sexual and reproductive health education (contraceptive methods, consistent condom use, prevention of vertical transmission and encouragement of voluntary HIV testing) can be a great advantage.

- The complexity of the issues involved in the dynamics of HIV risk behavior in both women and their partners seems evident. The stable relationship seems to legitimize the sexual relationship and thus detaches the woman from the action, leading to inconsistent condom use in the marital relationship. Many sexual partners refrain from using condoms in intramarital and extramarital relationships because of the cultural repertoire in which norms, values, stereotypes, power relations, feelings and meanings oppose the availability and capacity for safe sex. However, associating the expansion of the AIDS epidemic with "traditional" forms of sexual behavior, or with gender relations, without knowing the essence of sociocultural life in Angola, is an imposition on a strange reality.

- It is hoped that the results presented here can contribute to a reflection on the cultural patterns in Angolan society that can lead to the spread of HIV through sexual intercourse and that they can serve as a stimulus for further scientific work that makes it possible to adequately characterize the factors associated with sexual transmission in Angolan women.

BIBLIOGRAPHY CONSULTED

Galvao, Maria. T.G. et al. Uso do condom entre casais portadores ou não do HIV.In: Anais do III Congresso Brasileiro de Prevengao em DST/AIDS. 2.ed. Brasília: Ministério da Saúde: CN de DST/AIDS, 2000, p. 398-399.

UNAIDS AND WHO - Joint United Nations Program on HIV/AIDS (UNAIDS) and World Health Organization (WHO) 2009 . Situation of the AIDS epidemic. December 2009)

Brito AM, Castilho EA, Szwarcwald CL. AIDS and HIV infection in Brazil: a multifaceted epidemic. Rev Soc Bras Med Trop 2000; 34:207-17.

Neto, J.F.R; Lima, L.S.; Rocha, L. F.; Lima, J.S.; Santana, K.R.; Silveira, M.F. Perfil de adultos infectados pelo vírus da imunodeficiencia humana (HIV) em ambulatório de referencia em doengas sexualmente transmissíveis no norte de Minas Gerais- Rev Med Minas Gerais 2010; 20(1): 22-29,

Castilho and Chequer; Castilho, e. A. S. & Chequer, P.,. The AIDS epidemic in Brazil. In: A Epidemia de Aids no Brasil: Situagao e Tendencias (National Coordination of STD and AIDS of the Secretariat of Special Projects in Health, ed.), pp. 9-11, Brasília: Ministry of Health.1997

Castilho EA, Chequer P, Szwarcwld CL. AIDS in Brazil. In: Rouquayrol E, Almeida N (eds) Epidemiologia & Saúde. Editora Médica e Científica, Rio de Janeiro, p.271-284, 1999.

Olinto MTA, Galvao LW. Reproductive characteristics of women aged 15 to 49: comparative studies and august planning. Rev Saúde Pública 1999;33:64-72.

Parker R. Against AIDS: sexuality, intervention, politics. ABIA, Rio de Janeiro, Editora 34, Sao Paulo, 2000.

UNAIDS. Report on the global AIDS epidemic, 2004.

WHO, HIV infection prevention strategies, 1999. Available at: http://www.who.int, accessed on 28/10/05

Jones L, 1989. Women and HIV disease. Br J.Hosp.Med; 41: 526-38.

2.INLS - Instituto Nacional de Luta Contra a SIDA: Relatório de Actividades de 2005, Luanda, 2005. Ministry of Health - Republic of Angola.

. UNAIDS. Report on the global AIDS epidemic. Geneva; 2009.

Montagnier,N L. Virus and men - AIDS: its mechanisms and treatments. Rio de Janeiro. Jorge Zahar, 1995.

Brazil, Ministry of Health - Health Surveillance Secretariat - STD, AIDS and Viral Hepatitis Department. Epidemiological Bulletin - AIDS and STDs. Year VI - No. 1 - 27ª to 52ª - epidemiological weeks - 2008; Year VI - No. 1 - 01a to 26a - epidemiological weeks - January to June 2009. 2010.

Shisana O, Rehle T, Simbayi L, Parker W, Zuma K, Bhana A, et al, editors. South African national HIV prevalence, HIV Incidence, behavior and communication survey. Cape Town: HSRC Press; 2005

Szwarcwald CL, Bastos FI, Gravato N et al, 1998. The relationship of illicit drug consumption to HIVinfection among commercial sex workers (CSWs) in the city of Santos, Sao Paulo, Brazil. The International Journal of Drug

Policy 9:427-436.

.Muula, by Adamson S.. HIV Infection and AIDS Among Young Women in South Africa. Croat Med J 2008;49:423-435. www.cmj.hr ACCESSED 20 06 2010.

.Irffi, Guilherme ; Soares, Ricardo Brito; and DeSouza, Sergio Aquino - Socioeconomic, Demographic, Regional and Behavioral Factors that Influence Knowledge about HIV/AIDS . Brasília(DF), v.11, n.2, p.333-356, mai/ago 2010

. Santos, N. J. S.; Barbosa, R. M. ; Pinho, A.A.;Villele, W. V. ; Aidar, T.;. Filipe, E.M.V.. Contexts of vulnerability to HIV among Brazilian women. Cad. Saúde Pública, Rio de Janeiro, 25 Sup 2:S321-S333, 2009.

.Shisana O, Rehle T, Simbayi LC, Zuma K, Jooste S, Pillay-van-Wyk V,Mbelle N, Van Zyl J, Parker W, Zungu NP, Pezi S & the SABSSM III Implementation Team (2009) South African ational HIV prevalence, incidence, behavior and communication survey 2008: A turning tide among teenagers? Cape Town: HSRC Press2009

Silveira MF, Santos IS, Victora CG. Poverty, skin color and HIV infection: a case-control study from southern Brazil. AIDS Care 2008, 20:267-72.

.Varella, Rafael Brandao - Aspects of the AIDS epidemic in a medium-sized municipality in Rio de Janeiro, 2000-2004 . Rev Bras Epidemiol 2006; 9(4): 447-53.

Reis, C.T.; Czeresnia,D.; Barcellos, C.; Tassinari, W.S.- The internalization of the HIV/AIDS epidemic and the intermunicipal flow of hospital admissions in the Zona da Mata, Minas Gerais, Brazil: a spatial analysis. Cad. Saúde Pública vol.24 no.6 Rio de Janeiro June 2008 .

Brito AM, Castilho EA Szwarcwald CL . AIDS and HIV infection in Brazil: a multifaceted epidemic . Rev Soc Med Trop. 2001, 34 (2) :207 -17.

Rosenberg, P. S., 1995. Scope of the AIDS epidemic in the United States. Science, 270:1372-1375.

Greenland, S. LIEB, L. P.; Ford,W.& Kerndt, P. - Evidence for recent growth of the hiv epidemic among african-american men and younger male cohorts in los angeles county . Journal of acquired immune deficiency syndromes and human retrovirology, 11: 401-409.

Redinha, José. Distribuiçao Étnica de Angola, 8ª ed. Luanda, 1984

.Lukombo, Joao Baptista. Communities and community institutions in Angola in the post-war perspective: the case of the populations of Bakongo origin returning from the former Republic of Zaire and settled in the peri-urban fabric of Luanda". Ngola. Journal of Social Studies. Vol.I, n.º1. Luanda (1997), Associaçao dos Antropólogos e Sociólogos de Angola, pp. 251-278.

Fernandes, Joao; Ntondo, Zavoni. Angola: Peoples and Languages, Editorial Nzila. Luanda, 2002

Santos, C. A. Tambores incandescentes, corpos em êxtase- Técnicas e princípios bantus na performance ritual do Moçambique de Belém. PhD thesis presented to the Post-Graduate Program in Theatre at UNIRIO, under the supervision of Prof. Dr. Zeca Ligiéro. RIO DE JANEIRO, MARCH 2007 PNLS - National Program to Fight AIDS. Ministry of Health - Republic of Angola. Luanda, 1997.

.UNDP - United Nations Human Development Program: UNDP Human Development Report, 2007-2008.WHO Country Cooperation Strategy 2009-2013 ANGOLA - WHO 2009 ANGOLA PROFILE - WHO 2009

. Cassano, Conceiçâo; Frias, Luiz Armando de Medeiros; Valente, Joaquim Gonçalves Classification by occupation of AIDS cases in Brazil - 1995 - Cad. Saúde Pública v.16 supl.1 Rio de Janeiro 2000.

. Konopka, C K; Beck, S T; Wiggers, D; Kieslich da Silva, A; Diehl, F P; Santos, F G. Clinical and epidemiological profile of HIV-infected pregnant women in a service in southern Brazil. Rev. Bras. Ginecol. Obstet. vol.32 no.4 Rio de Janeiro Apr. 2010

. SANTOS , S. M. S. e Oliveira, M. L. F.- (Com)vivendo com a Aids: perfil dos portadores de HIV/Aids na regiâo Noroeste do Estado do Paraná, 19892005 Acta Scientiarum. Health Sciences Maringá, v. 32, n. 1, p. 51-56, 2009.

.Heilborn, M. L. (org.), 1999, "Sexualidade - o olhar das ciências sociais", Jorge Zahar Editor.

.Ribeiro, J. T. Evoluçâo da Populaçâo de Angola 1940-2005. Retrieved June 17, 2007b

Santos NJS, Buchalla CM, Filipe EMV, Bugamelli L, Garcia S, Paiva V. HIV-positive women, reproduction and sexuality. Rev Saúde Pública 2002; 36: 12-23.

.JUNIOR, MANUEL GARCIA. Saudade- COINGRA- Companhia Industrial Gráfica dos Açores, Ld.ª , Parue Industrial da Ribeira Grande, 1984. Luanda, 1995

Machava, Joaquim Rafael. The Poverty Situation in Mozambique: Regional Differences and Main Challenges. Geographical Studies, Rio Claro, 5(1): 27-46, 2007 (ISSN 1678-698X).

Parpinelli, M.A; Faúndes, A.; Cecatti,J.G.; Pereira,B.G.; Júnior,R.P.; Amaral,E. Analysis of Avoidable Mortality in Women of Reproductive Age Rev. Bras. Ginecol. Obstet. vol.22 no.9 Rio de Janeiro Oct. 2000

.Joâo, Paulo. Approach to HIV/AIDS transmission in sex workers in Luanda - Angola - Africa: A challenge called Angola. Master's dissertation presented to the Faculty of Medical Sciences, State University of Campinas, for the degree of Master in Collective Health. Campinas, 2005.

Vitor da Silva, B - Socio-demographic Profile and Health Conditions of the Population of Guinea-Bissau in 2002. Dissertation presented to the Postgraduate Course in Demography at the Center for Development and Regional Planning of the Faculty of Economic Sciences of the Federal University of Minas Gerais, Belo Horizonte, MG UFMG/ CEDEPLAR 2005.

Brazil. Ministry of Health. Theoretical and referential framework. Sexual and reproductive health of adolescents and young people. Brasília: Ministry of Health; 2006

Lopes, F.; Buchalla, C.M.; Ayres, J.R.C.M. Black and non-black women and vulnerability to HIV/AIDS in the state of Sáo Paulo, Brazil Rev. Saúde.

AYRES, J. R. C. M., 1994. Epidemiologia sem números: Outras reflexoes sobre a ciencia epidemiológica, a propósito da AIDS. In: Seminar on the Social Epidemiology of AIDS, *Proceedings,* pp. 8-19, Rio de Janeiro: ABIA/IMS-UERJ.

SWEAT, M. D. & DENNISON, J. A., 1995. Reducing HIV incidence in developing countries with structural and environmental interventions. *AIDS,* 9 (Suppl. A): S251-S257.

TAWIL, O.; VERSTER, A. & O'REILLY, K. R., 1995. Enabling approaches for HIV/AIDS prevention: Can we modify the environment and minimize the risk? *AIDS,* 9:1299-1306.

TURSHEN, M., 1995. Response: Societal instability in international perspective: Relevance to HIV/AIDS Prevention. In: *Assessing the Social and Behavioral Science Base for HIV/AIDS Prevention and Intervention* [Workshop Summary], pp. 117-128, Washington, D.C.: National Academy Press.

AGGLETON, P., 1996. Global priorities for HIV/AIDS intervention research. *International Journal of Sexually Transmitted Diseases and AIDS,* 7 (Suppl. 2):13-16.

CARAEL, M.; BUVÉ, A. & AWUSABO-ASARE, K., 1997. The making of HIV epidemics: What are the driving forces? *AIDS,* 11 (Suppl. B):S23-S31.

PARKER, Richard and CAMARGO JR., Kenneth Rochel de. Poverty and HIV/AIDS: anthropological and sociological aspects. Cad. Saúde Pública, Rio de Janeiro, 16(Suppl. 1):89-102, 2000.

UNAIDS. Report on the global AIDS epidemic. Geneva; 2009.

UNAIDS AND WHO - Joint United Nations Program on HIV/AIDS (UNAIDS) and World Health Organization (WHO) 2009 . Situation of the AIDS epidemic. UNAIDS/09.36S / JC1700S (Spanish version, December 2009).

INLS - National Institute for the Fight Against AIDS: 2005 Activity Report, Luanda, 2005. Ministry of Health - Republic of Angola.

PAULO, JOÁO. Approach to HIV/AIDS transmission in sex workers in Luanda - Angola - Africa: A challenge called Angola. Master's dissertation presented to the Faculty of Medical Sciences, State University of Campinas, for the degree of Master in Collective Health. Campinas, 2004

PRATA, BY NDOLA; VAHIDNIA, FARNAZ; FRASER, ASHLEY - Gender and Relationship Differences in Condom Use Among 15-24-Year-Olds in Angola .

International Family Planning Perspectives Gender and Relationship Differences in Condom Use Among Angolan Youth. Volume 31, Number 4, December 2005.

MONTEIRO, SIMONE - STD/AIDS prevention in Portuguese-speaking Africa: a review of the recent literature in the social sciences and health.

Cadernos de Saúde Pública, Rio de Janeiro, 25 (3) :680-686, Mar, 2009

LOFORTE, A. M. - Inequalities and values in reproductive health. La vulnerabilidad de las mujeres en un contexto de feminización del sida IN : Degregori, Maria Cristina Álvarez ; Reguillo, Esther Leandro ; DiGiacomo, Susan; Guidoum, Yamina - Mulher, Sida y Acesso a La Salud em Africa Subsahariana: Enfoque desde las ciencias socialies. Medicus Mundi Catalunya. Barcelona February 2007 .

DEGREGORI, MARIA CRISTINA ÁLVAREZ ; REGUILLO, ESTHER LEANDRO ; DIGIACOMO, SUSAN; GUIDOUM, YAMINA - Women, AIDS and Access to Health in Sub-Saharan Africa: An Approach from the Social Sciences. Medicus Mundi Catalunya. Barcelona February 2007 .

SAFFIOTI HIB. Rearticulating gender and social class. In: Costa AO, Bruschini C (org.). Uma questão de genero. Rio de Janeiro/Sao Paulo: Rosa dos Tempos/Fundagao Carlos Chagas; 1992: 183-215.

SILVA, C.M.; VARGENS, O. M. da COSTA. Women's perception of their vulnerability to STD/HIV infection. Revista da Escola de Enfermagem da USP Rev. esc. enferm. USP vol.43 no.2 Sao Paulo June 2009.

BUCHALLA CM, PAIVA V. - From understanding social vulnerability to a multidisciplinary approach. Rev Saúde Pública. 2002;36 (4):117-9.

SALDANHA AAW. - Vulnerability and coping constructions of HIV seropositivity by infected women in a stable relationship [thesis]. Sao Paulo: Ribeirao Preto Faculty of Philosophy, Sciences and Letters, University of Sao Paulo; 2005.

WERNECK J. - The vulnerability of black women. Jornal da Rede Saúde [periodical on the Internet]. 2001 Mar [cited 2005 Sep 14];(23).

KALIPENI, E, GHOSH, J, AWIRE-VALHMU, L M - The multiple dimensions of vulnerability in the face of the hiv/aids epidemic in Africa: a sociological perspective the conceptual framework of vulnerability in degregori, m c a; reguillo, e l; digiacomo, s; guidoum, y- women, aids and access to health in sub-saharan africa: an approach from the social sciences. mogambique, february 2007.

RUSHING, WILLIAM A., 1995 The AIDS Epidemic: Social Dimensions of an Infectious Disease. Boulder, Colorado: Westview Press.

Shannon, Gary W., Gerald F. Pyle, y Rashid Bashshur, 1991 The Geography of AIDS: Origins and Course of an Epidemic. New York: Guilford Press.

OPPONG, JOSEPH R., Y EZEKIEL KALIPENI, 1999 - A Cross-Cultural Perspective on AIDS in Africa: A Response to Rushing. African Rural and Urban Studies 3(2):91-112

GARCIA-MORENO C, JANSEN HA, ELLSBERG M, HEISE L, WATTS C. WHO Multicountry study on women's health and domestic violence against women - initial results on prevalence, health outcomes and women's responses. Geneva: World Health Organization; 2005.

SCHRAIBER LILIA BLIMA, LATORRE MARIA DO ROSÁRIO DIAS O, FRANÇA JR IVAN, SEGRI NEUBER JOSÉ, D'OLIVEIRA ANA FLÁVIA PIRES LUCAS. Validity of the WHO VAW STUDY instrument for estimating gender-based violence against women. Rev. Saúde Pública, 2010; 44(4): 658-666.

SCHRAIBER LB, D'OLIVEIRA AFPL, FRANÇA JR I, DINIZ S, PORTELLA AP, LUDERMIR AB, et al. Prevalence of intimate partner violence against women in regions of Brazil. Rev Saude Publica. 2007.

BARNEY COEN AND JAMES TRUSSELL- Preventing and mitigating aids in sub-Saharan Afric- Research and data priorities for the social and behavioral sciences. National Academy Press Washintogton, D.C. 1996. - USAID.gov 08 08 2010.

FONSECA, F. E LUCAS, M. C. L. Sexuality, health and contexts: influence of culture and ethnicity on sexual behavior - dossier: multiculturalism. Rev Port Clin Geral 2009;25:65-72.

DIAS S, MATOS MG, GONÇALVES A. Sexual behavior: self-reports in a migrant community. Rev Port Pedagogia 2001; XXXV-2: 137--54.

BRADBY H,WILLIAMS R.- Behaviours and expectations in relation to sexual intercourse among 18-20 year old Asian and non-Asians. Sex Transm Infect 1999 Jun; 75 (3): 162-7.

JUNIOR, MANUEL GARCIA. Saudade- COINGRA- Companhia Industrial Gráfica dos Açores, Ld.ª , Parue Industrial da Ribeira Grande, 1984. Luanda, 1995.

MAKINWA-ADEBUSOYE, PAULINA. Socio-cultural factors influencing fertility in sub-Saharan Africa. United Nations Population Bulletin, pages 46 to 47, 2002.

PEN- National Strategic Plan for Sexually Transmitted Diseases, HIV and AIDS in Angola, July 1999.Ministério da Saúde - Angola.

ANGOLA - UNDP - United Nations Human Development Program - past, present and future. Angola, 2001.

ALLEN S, LINDAN C, CHEN RUNDLE A, et al. HIV in urban Rwanda: demographic and behavioral correlates in a representative sample of childbearing women. JAMA 1991;266:1657-1663.

UNITED NATIONS Distr.: General. November 7, 2002. Committee on the Elimination of Discrimination against Women. Consideration of reports submitted by States parties under article 18 of the Convention on the Elimination of All Forms of Discrimination against Women. Combined initial, second and third periodic reports of States parties. Angola*. AVAILABLE AT http://daccess-dds- y.un.org/doc/UNDOC

SCHRAIBER LB, D'OLIVEIRA AFPL, Couto MT. Violence and Health: theoretical, methodological and ethical contributions from studies of violence against women. Cad Saude Publica. 2009;25(Supl 2):205-16.

Breith J. Mujer, trabajo y salud. Quito: CEAS, 1994;vol 1:17,304-7.

REVISTA CUBANA DE SAUDE PUBLICA. http://bvs.sld.cu

HEISE, L., 1994. Violence Against Women: The Hidden Health Burden. Report Prepared for the World Bank. (Mimeo.) (Manuscript published under the same title in the series World Bank Discussion Papers 255, Washington, D.C.: World Bank, 1994).

CARDOSO, N. M. (1997b). Women and abuse. In M. Strey (Org.). Mulher: Estudos de género (pp. 127-138). Sao Leopoldo: Unisinos.

LAIRD, J. (2002). Women's secrets: Women's silence. In E. Imber-Black (Org.). Secrets in the family and family therapy (pp. 245-268). Porto Alegre: Artes Médicas.

MASON, M. J. (2002). Shame: A reservoir for secrets in the family. In E. Imber-Black (Org.). Secrets in the family and in family therapy (pp. 40-56). Porto Alegre: Artes Médicas.

NARVAZ, M. G. and KOLLER, S. H.- Women victims of domestic violence: Understanding subjectivities that are subjected. PSICO, Porto Alegre, PUCRS, v. 37, n. 1, pp. 7-13, jan./abr. 2006

Dunkle KL, Jewkes RK, Brown HC, et al. Genderbased violence, relationship power, and risk of HIV infection in women attending antenatal clinics in South Africa. Lancet 2004;363:1415-1421.

Jewkes R, Levin J, Penn-Kekana L. Risk factors for domestic violence: fi ndings from a South African crosssectional study. *Soc Sci Med.* 2002;55(9):1603-17. DOI:10.1016/S0277-9536(01)00294-5.

JEWKES, R.K; DUNKLE, K; NDUNA, M; SHAI, N. Intimate partner violence, relationship power inequity, and incidence of HIV infection in young women in South Africa: a cohort study. The Lancet, Volume 376, Issue 9734, Pages 41 - 48, July 3, 2010.

ALLEN S, LINDAN C, CHEN RUNDLE A, et al. HIV in urban Rwanda: demographic and behavioral correlates in a representative sample of childbearing women. JAMA 1991;266:1657-1663.

Mnm COHEN MS. HAART and Prevention of HIV Transmission. Conference Report. Medscape HIV/AIDS 8(2), 2002.©2002 Medscape.

UNAIDS. AIDS Epidemic Update: December 2007

SINGER M, 1994. AIDS and the health crisis of the U.S. urban poor; the perspective of critical medical anthropology. Social Science and Medicine 39: 93148.

O'DONNELL L, O'DONNELL CR Y STUEVE A. Early sexual initiation and subsequent sex-related risk among urban minority youth: The reach for health study. Fam Plan Perspect. 2001;33:268-275.

PETTIFOR AE, VAN DER STRATEN A, DUNBAR MS, SHIBOSKI SC Y PADIAN NS. Early age of first sex: A risk factor for HIV infection among women in Zimbabwe. AIDS. 2004;18:1435-1442.;

BEADNELL B, MORRISON DM, WILSDON A, WELLS EA, MUROWCHICK E, HOPPE M et al. Condom use, frequency of sex, and number of partners: Multidimensional characterization of adolescent sexual risk taking. J Sex Res. 2005;42:192-202.

SILVEIRA, M.F.; BÉRIA, J.U.; HORTA,B.L.; TOMASI,E. Self-perception of risk for STD/AIDS Rev Saúde Pública 2002;36(6):670-7 677

SILVA, C.M.; VARGENS, O. M. DA COSTA. Women's perception of their vulnerability to STD/HIV infection. Revista da Escola de Enfermagem da USP Rev. esc. enferm. USP vol.43 no.2 São Paulo June 2009.

BUCHALLA CM, PAIVA V. From understanding social vulnerability to a multidisciplinary approach. Rev Saúde Pública. 2002;36 (4):117-9.

SALDANHA AAW. Vulnerability and coping constructs of HIV seropositivity by infected women in a stable relationship [thesis]. São Paulo: Ribeirão Preto School of Philosophy, Sciences and Letters, University of São Paulo; 2005.

WERNECK J. Vulnerability of black women. Jornal da Rede Saúde [periodical on the Internet]. 2001 Mar [cited 2005 Sep 14];(23). Available from: http://www. antroposmoderno. com/antro-articulo.php?idarticulo=309.

SEIDMAN SN, MOSHER WD, ARAL SO. Predictors of high-risk behavior in unmarried Americanwomen: adolescent environment as risk factor. J Adolesc Health 1994;15:126-32.

ALAN GUTTMACHER INSTITUTE. Toward a new world: the sexual and reproductive lives of young women. New York: The Alan Guttmacher Institute; 1998.

OLINTO MT A, GALVÄO LW. Reproductive characteristics of women aged 15 to 49: comparative studies and aedes planning. Rev Saúde Pública 1999;33:64-72.

SHEPHERD J, WESTON R, PEERSMAN G, NAPULI IZ. Cervical cancer and sexual lifestyle: a systematic reviewof health education interventions targeted at women. Health Educ Res 2000;15:681-94.

SANTOS, SONIA MARIA SOARES DOS E OLIVEIRA, MAGDA LÚCIA FÉLIX - (Com)vivendo com a Aids: perfil dos portadores de HIV/Aids na regiäo Noroeste do Estado do Paraná, 1989-2005 Acta Scientiarum. Health Sciences Maringá, v. 32, n. 1, p. 51-56, 2009.

SAFFIOTI HIB. Rearticulating gender and social class. In: Costa AO, Bruschini C (org.). Uma questão de genero. Rio de Janeiro/Säo Paulo: Rosa dos Tempos/Fundaeäo Carlos Chagas; 1992: 183-215.

QUINN SC. AIDS and the African-American woman: The triple burden of race, class and gender. Health Educ Q 1993; 20(3): 305-20.

VILLELA W. Women, violence and AIDS: exploring interfaces. In: Nilo A, organizer. Women, violence and AIDS. Recife: GESTOS - Soropositividade, Comunicaeäo & Genero; 2008. p. 107-26.

JIMENEZ AL, GOTLIEB SLD, HARDY E, ZANEVELD LJD. Prevention of sexually transmitted diseases in women: association with socioeconomic and demographic variables. Cad Saúde Pública 2001;17:55-62.

SEIDMAN SN, MOSHER WD, ARAL SO. Women with multiple sexual partners: United States, 1988. Am J Public Health 1992;82:1388-94

DAVIS, KR, WELLER SC. The effectiveness of condoms in reducing heterosexual transmission of HIV. Family Planning Perspectives 1999; 31(6):272-79

CHIN D. HIV-related sexual risk assessment among Asian/Pacific Islander American women: an inductive model. Soc Sci Med 1999; 49:241-51

PRAÇA NS, GUALDA DMR. Risk of HIV infection: how women living in a favela perceive themselves in the chain of transmission of the virus. Ver Latinoam Enfermagem 2003; 11:14-20.

HEBLING EM, GUIMARÃES IRF. Women and AIDS: gender relations and condom use with steady partners. Cad Saúde Pública 2004; 20:1211-8.

AMORIM MM, ANDRADE NA. Affective-sexual relationships and prevention of sexually transmitted infections and AIDS among women in the municipality of Vitória -ES. Psicol Estud 2006; 11:331-9.

SANTOS, C.O E IRIART, J.A.B Meanings and practices associated with the risk of contracting HIV in the sexual itineraries of women from a popular neighborhood in Salvador, Bahia, Brazil Cad. Saúde Pública, Rio de Janeiro, 23(12):2896-2905, dec, 2007.

ALVES RN, KOVÁCS MJ, STALL R, PAIVA V. Psychosocial factors and HIV infection in women, Maringá, PR. Rev Saúde Pública. 2002;36 Supl 4:329

THIENGO MA, OLIVEIRA DC, RODRIGUES BMRD. Social representations of HIV/AIDS among adolescents: implications for nursing care. Rev Esc Enferm USP. 2005; 39(1):68-76.

GIACOMOZZI, A. I, CAMARGO, B.C. Eu confio no meu marido: estudo da representação social de mulheres com parceiro fixo sobre prevençâo da AIDS. In: Psicologia: Teoria e prática, Sâo Paulo, 2004, n. 6, v. 1, p. 31-44.

NASCIMENTO AMG, BARBOSA CS, MEDRADO B. Women in Camaragibe: social representation of female vulnerability in times of AIDS. Rev Bras Saúde Mater Infant. 2005;5

SILVA, C.M.; VARGENS, O. M. DA COSTA. Women's perception of their vulnerability to STD/HIV infection. Revista da Escola de Enfermagem da USP Rev. esc. enferm. USP vol.43 no.2 Sâo Paulo June 2009.

GIACOMOZZI AI, CAMARGO BV. Trust in partners and protection against HIV: a study of social representations. Master's thesis. Postgraduate Program in Psychology, Federal University of Santa Catarina - Florianópolis. 2004. Cited on April 18, 2006.

SAFFIOTI HIB. Rearticulating gender and social class. In: Costa AO, Bruschini C (org.). Uma questão de gênero. Rio de Janeiro/Sâo Paulo: Rosa dos Tempos/Fundaçâo Carlos Chagas; 1992: 183-215.

GOGNA, MÓNICA. Contributions to rethinking STD prevention. In. II Seminar on reproductive health in times of AIDS. ABIA: Program of Studies and Research in Gender, Sexuality and Health - IMS/UERJ, 1997. (op. cit. p. 55-6)

BUCHALLA CM, PAIVA V. From understanding social vulnerability to a multidisciplinary approach. Rev Saúde Pública. 2002;36 (4):117-9.

SALDANHA AAW. Vulnerability and coping constructions of HIV seropositivity by infected women in a stable relationship [thesis]. Sao Paulo: Ribeirao Preto School of Philosophy, Sciences and Letters, University of Sao Paulo; 2005.

SIMOES-BARBOSA RH. AIDS & reproductive health: new challenges. In: Giffin K, Costa SH, organizers. Reproductive health issues. Rio de Janeiro:

Editora Fiocruz; 1999. p. 281-98.

Worth D. Sexual decisionmaking and Aids: why condom promotion among vulnerable women is likely to fail. Studies in Family Planning 1989;20(6):297-307.

Pivnick A. HIV infection and the meaning of condoms. Culture and Medical Psychiatry 1993;17:431-53.

UNAIDS, 2006 - JOINT UNITED NATION PROGRAMME ON HIV/AIDS (UNAIDS) - Alcohol Use and Sexual Risk Behavior: A Cross-Cultural Study in Eight Countries, 2006.

BENOTSCH, E.G.; PINKERTON, S.D.; DYATLOV, R.V.; DIFRANCEISCO, W.; SMIRNOVA, T.S.; DUDKO, V.Y., et al. - HIV risk behavior in male and female Russian sexually transmitted disease clinic patients. Int J Behav Med 13(1): 26-33, 2006.

CARDOSO, LUCIANA ROBERTA DONOLA; MALBERGIER, ANDRÉ; FIGUEIREDO, TATHIANA FERNANDES BISCUOLA. Alcohol consumption as a risk factor for the transmission of STDs/HIV/AIDS. Rev. psiquiatr. clín. vol.35 suppl.1 Sao Paulo 2008.

MALOW, R.M.; DÉVIEUX, J.G.; JENNINGS, T.; LUCENKO, B.A.; KALICHMAN, S.C. - Substance-abusing adolescents at varying levels of HIV risk: psychosocial characteristics, drug use, and sexual behavior. J Subst Abuse 13(1-2): 103-117. 2001

BACHANAS, P.J.; MORRIS, M.K.; LEWIS-GESS, J.K.; SARETT-CUASAY, E.J.; FLORES, A.L.; SIRL, K.S., et al. - Psychological adjustment, substance use, HIV knowledge, and risky sexual behavior in at-risk minority females: developmental differences during adolescence. Journal of Pediatric Psychology vol. 27(4): 373-384, 2002.

DICLEMENTE, R.J.; WINGOOD, G.M.; SIONEAN, C.; CROSBY, R.; HARRINGTON, K.; DAVIES, S., et al. - Association of adolescents history of sexually transmitted disease (STD) and their current high-risk behavior and STD status: a case for intensifying clinic-based prevention efforts. Sex Transm Dis 29(9): 503-509, 2002

GRIFFIN, K.W; BOTVIN, G.J.; NICHOLS, T.R. - Effects of a school-based drug abuse prevention program for adolescents on HIV risk behavior in young adulthood. Prev Sci 7(1): 103-112, 2006.

LIU, A.; KILMARX, P.; JENKINS, R.A.; MANOPAIBOON, C.; MOCK, P.A.; JEEYAPUNT, S., et al. - Sexual initiation, substance use, and sexual behavior and knowledge among vocational students in northern Thailand. Int Fam Plan Perspect 32(3): 126-135, 2006.

ROBERTS, S.T.; KENNEDY, B.L. - Why are young college women not using condoms? Their perceived risk, drug use, and developmental vulnerability may provide important clues to sexual risk. Arch Psychiatr Nurs 20(1): 32-40, 2006.

MSUYA, S.E.; MBIZVO, E.; HUSSAIN, A.; URIYO, J.; SAM, N.E.; STRAY-PEDERSEN B. - HIV among pregnant women in Moshi Tanzania: the role of sexual behavior, male partner characteristics and sexually transmitted infections. AIDS Res Ther 3: 27, 2006.

MUULA, BY ADAMSON S.. HIV Infection and AIDS Among Young Women in South Africa. Croat Med J 2008;49:423-435.

UNAIDS AND WHO - Joint United Nations Program on HIV/AIDS (UNAIDS) and World Health Organization (WHO) 2009 . Situation of the AIDS epidemic. UNAIDS/09.36S / JC1700S (Spanish version, December 2009).

Khobotlo M et al. (2009). *Lesotho: HIV prevention response and modes of transmission analysis*. Maseru, Lesotho National AIDS Commission.

MAKINWA-ADEBUSOYE, PAULINA. Socio-cultural factors influencing fertility in sub-Saharan Africa. United Nations Population Bulletin, pages 46 to 47, 2002.

GIR, ELUCIR E GESSOLO, FABIANA - AIDS knowledge and changes in professional attitudes. USP Nursing School. V 32 n°2 p 91-100, August 1998

BASTOS FI, CUNHA CB, BERTONI N. Use of psychoactive substances and contraceptive methods by the Brazilian urban population, 2005. Rev Saúde Pública 2008; 42 Suppl 1:118-26.

WALQUE, D. (2006). Who gets AIDS and how? The determinants of HIV infection and sexual behaviors in Burkina Faso, Cameroon, Ghana, Kenya and Tanzania. World Bank in its series Policy Research Working Paper Series 3844

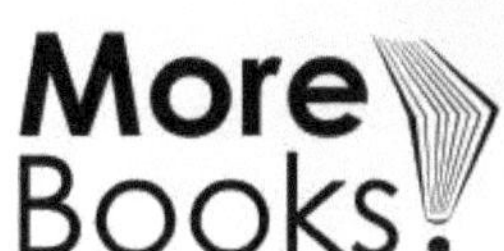

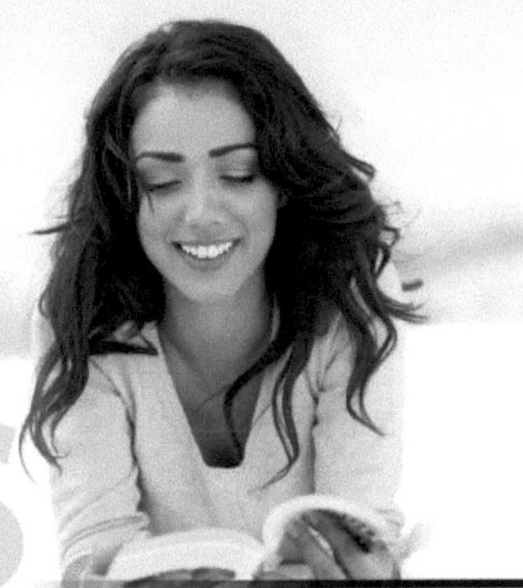

Buy your books fast and straightforward online - at one of world's fastest growing online book stores! Environmentally sound due to Print-on-Demand technologies.

Buy your books online at
www.morebooks.shop

Kaufen Sie Ihre Bücher schnell und unkompliziert online – auf einer der am schnellsten wachsenden Buchhandelsplattformen weltweit! Dank Print-On-Demand umwelt- und ressourcenschonend produziert.

Bücher schneller online kaufen
www.morebooks.shop

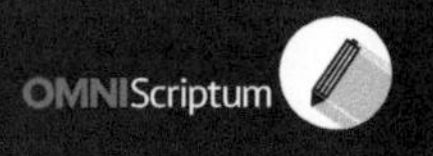

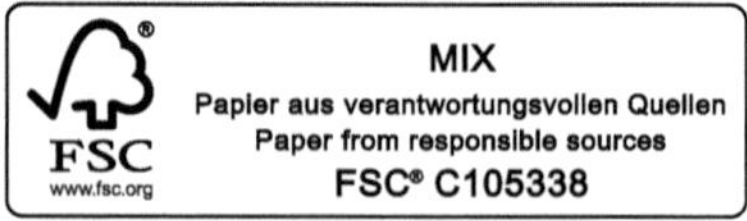

Printed by Books on Demand GmbH, Norderstedt / Germany